# 101 Tips for Aging Well with Diabetes

David B. Kelley, MD

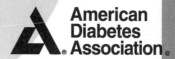

American Diabetes Association.

*Director, Book Publishing,* John Fedor; *Book Acquisitions,* Sherrye Landrum; *Editor,* Abe Ogden; *Production Manager,* Peggy M. Rote; *Composition,* Circle Graphics, Inc.; *Cover Design,* Wickham & Associates, Inc.; *Printer,* Transcontinental Printing

Printed in Canada

1 3 5 7 9 10 8 6 4 2

The suggestions and information contained in this publication are generally consistent with the *Clinical Practice Recommendations* and other policies of the American Diabetes Association, but they do not represent the policy or position of the Association or any of its boards or committees. Reasonable steps have been taken to ensure the accuracy of the information presented. However, the American Diabetes Association cannot ensure the safety or efficacy of any product or service described in this publication. Individuals are advised to consult a physician or other appropriate health care professional before undertaking any diet or exercise program or taking any medication referred to in this publication. Professionals must use and apply their own professional judgment, experience, and training and should not rely solely on the information contained in this publication before prescribing any diet, exercise, or medication. The American Diabetes Association—its officers, directors, employees, volunteers, and members—assumes no responsibility or liability for personal or other injury, loss, or damage that may result from the suggestions or information in this publication.

⊗ The paper in this publication meets the requirements of the ANSI Standard Z39.48-1992 (permanence of paper).

ADA titles may be purchased for business or promotional use or for special sales. For information, please write to Lee Romano Sequeira, Special Sales & Promotions, at the address below.

American Diabetes Association
1701 North Beauregard Street
Alexandria, Virginia 22311

**Library of Congress Cataloging-in-Publication Data**

Kelley, David B.
    101 tips for aging well with diabetes / David B. Kelley.
        p. cm.
    Includes index.
    ISBN 1-58040-039-6
        1. Diabetes in old age—Popular works. 2. Diabetes—Popular works. I. Title: One hundred tips for aging well with diabetes. II. Title.

RC660.75 .K45 2001
616.4'62—dc21                                                    2001022959

# 101 TIPS FOR AGING WELL WITH DIABETES

# TABLE OF CONTENTS

# PREFACE

*How old would you be if you didn't know how*
*old you are?*

−Satchell Paige

Should there be a book about aging well with diabetes? Yes, just as there should be a book about aging well in general. No matter how old you are, what happens today is something you've never done before. Wouldn't you like to do it the very best way you can? Look at it this way: aging begins the day we're born. We're here to grow and learn.

Diabetes always adds a new dimension to people's health responsibilities. Diabetes that happens in later life is usually different from the diabetes of youth, but the challenges are the same. It's important to focus on aging well with diabetes because diabetes can have a great impact on your overall health, and your overall health will impact your diabetes. You can tame diabetes and make the impact a positive one—the future is in your hands.

If your date of birth is far distant, you have experience and authority and seasoning and discipline and wisdom. With these qualities, you are well equipped to grasp the significance and importance of the lessons that diabetes is bringing to you.

# Chapter 1
# GETTING ORGANIZED

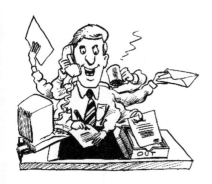

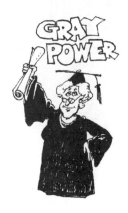

*A*s I age, how do I take care of my *diabetes?*

▼
## TIP:

Diabetes can have a large impact on your life no matter how old you are, but with some organization and a bit of discipline to be proud of, it won't stop you from living the life you want to live. There is a plan for living with diabetes and by following it, you're on your way to a happier, longer life. The main points of this plan are:

- Acceptance and a positive attitude
- Education—at diagnosis and again every few years
- Eating in a healthy way—more fresh vegetables and fruit
- Exercising daily
- Achieving a desirable weight—even 20 pounds lighter helps
- Checking glucose levels at home
- Using medications for diabetes, if needed
- Working with health care professionals who have training in diabetes
- Getting support of family, friends, and community

Learn the skills of diabetes management. You are the expert on you. It is up to you to adapt the plan to fit your lifestyle and your needs.

*I* *was never good in school and that*
*was years ago. Am I smart enough*
*to get educated about diabetes?*

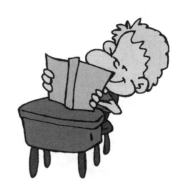

▼
# TIP:

Yes. It doesn't take book smarts to learn about diabetes. Here's an example. In his mid-40s, Kurt had his pancreas removed to avoid pancreatic cancer. The operation caused full-blown, insulin-dependent diabetes. Kurt also has a mental development disorder. He lives alone with supervision. His surgeons assumed that a detailed diabetes treatment plan would be too complicated and sent him home with a simpler plan. Unfortunately, the plan didn't give him enough information, and he was in blood sugar chaos.

Kurt knew his only chance for stable health was through diabetes education and fine-tuning his care plan. He rose to the challenge and has learned well. His HbA1c levels are great, and he seldom has low blood sugars because he heads them off before they happen. His physician ranks him at the head of the class.

It doesn't take smarts. It takes you realizing that education can help you with your diabetes. Then it takes desire, a teacher, and support from your health care provider. You can do it if you want to.

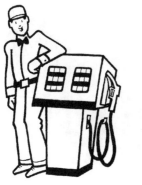

# *W*hat is diabetes?

▼
**TIP:**

Diabetes is diagnosed when you have high levels of glucose (sugar) in your blood. Something goes wrong in getting energy from the food you eat, a process called metabolism. Food is broken down to glucose, and the glucose goes into the bloodstream to get to all the cells. Insulin, a hormone produced by your pancreas, is the key that unlocks the door to the cells.

When insulin can't do its job (type 2 diabetes), or when your pancreas can't produce insulin (type 1 diabetes), the cells can't get the glucose. You continue to eat—in fact you will feel that you are starving (your cells are)—but glucose just continues to build up in your bloodstream. Then you have high blood sugar levels all the time—diabetes.

Gestational diabetes occurs in some women only when they are pregnant. People with type 2 who lose weight and start exercising can bring their blood sugar levels back to normal, so it may appear they are healed. But their diabetes is just under very good control. Good control prevents or postpones the complications of diabetes from developing and makes you feel good every day.

*W*hat are the differences between type 1 diabetes and type 2 diabetes?

▼
## TIP:

They have one thing in common—high blood sugar—and treatments are similar. People with type 1 diabetes do not make any insulin, so they must have insulin by injection to live. Type 1 diabetes tends to occur in younger people and comes on rather quickly. Type 1 is caused when insulin-producing beta cells in the pancreas are mistakenly destroyed by the immune system.

Type 2 diabetes is the most common type of diabetes. The body becomes resistant to its own insulin, which means it must produce more. Over time the pancreas may just wear out, which is why it takes time to detect type 2 diabetes—it happens gradually. People who develop it are often quite overweight. Weight loss and exercise improve blood glucose levels, and many people also take diabetes pills. As time passes, about 40 % of people with type 2 need insulin injections to control their blood glucose levels, especially if their blood glucose has been uncontrolled for a long time.

Meal planning and exercise are part of the diabetes care plan for both types of diabetes.

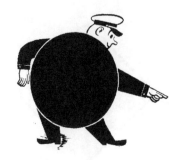

*My doctor told me I have borderline diabetes. What does this mean?*

▼
## TIP:

It means you have diabetes. Borderline diabetes or a "touch of sugar" or any term like that means that you have diabetes—and your provider should be more up to date. If your blood glucose levels are above the cutoff point, you have diabetes. The problem is, when your blood glucose is just approaching the cutoff level, you are still at risk for the same health problems of someone who has diabetes—heart disease, nerve damage, kidney damage, and stroke.

Unfortunately, many patients and physicians don't treat borderline cases as serious, and this can lead to serious problems later on. If your blood glucose levels are close to the diabetic levels, talk to your health care practitioner about what steps to take right now to get your blood glucose nearer normal. Losing some weight—even 10 to 20 pounds—makes a considerable improvement in your blood glucose level. And exercise is the magic pill we're all looking for—try it, too. Taking action now can prevent all kinds of complications down the road.

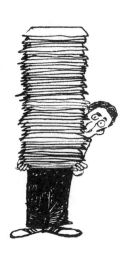

*I*'m in my 70s, and I just got diabetes.
How many other people my age have it?

▼
## TIP:

More than 16 million people in the United States have diabetes, with that number steadily increasing. The number of diabetes cases is about equal between men and women and increases with each passing decade of life. As you can see, more than 30 % of people over the age of 60 have diabetes or impaired fasting glucose—meaning they have higher than normal blood glucose levels but not as high as the level for diabetes. Unfortunately, only 10 million of these people are diagnosed and under treatment, and of those 10 million, only 5 million are getting the best care!

| Age | Percent of Population with Diabetes and/or Impaired Fasting Glucose |
| --- | --- |
| 20 to 39 | 5 % |
| 40 to 49 | 13 % |
| 50 to 59 | 20 % |
| 60 or above | 30 % or more |

Your ethnic background also makes a difference. African Americans and Latinos are almost twice as likely to get diabetes.

You are definitely not alone!

# Will I get long-term complications of diabetes?

▼
**TIP:**

There is no definite answer to this. Many of the complications often linked with diabetes are the same complications that come to people with advancing age, such as poor circulation or blurry vision. Others are unique to diabetes, such as retinopathy and kidney damage. Most parts of the body can be affected by high blood sugar levels over a long period of time. Too much of anything is not good, and as time passes, high blood sugar causes chemical and structural injury to delicate tissues, especially in blood vessels and nerves.

The best way to prevent complications is to keep your blood sugar under control—nearer to normal levels. Even if you already have some complications, you can slow them down and, sometimes, reverse the damage by getting your blood glucose under better control. This is your best defense against complications. Figuring out how to manage your diabetes better is an investment in time and energy that pays big dividends by making you feel better day to day and keeping you healthier over the long run.

*D*oes having diabetes mean I'm going to have a shorter life expectancy?

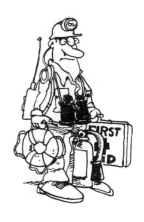

▼
## TIP:

No, not necessarily. Fifty years ago, it was thought that if you had type 1 diabetes, you'd barely make middle age, and if you had mature-onset type 2, you were nearing the end. Many people have received their 50-year medals from the Eli Lilly Company, celebrating fifty years with diabetes and putting to rest the fears about life expectancy. The future is bright for people with diabetes. Technologies to help you control your blood sugar are much better, medications are better, treatments are more effective, and we know a lot more about the disease than in the past.

Still, the choice is up to you. All of the advancements in diabetes care don't mean anything if you're not committed to proper blood glucose management. If you don't take care of your diabetes, your diabetes will take care of you in ways you'd probably not prefer.

Many people live with diabetes for 40, 50, even 70 years, but it's because they stay committed to their care. How committed are you?

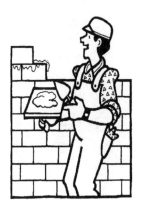

*A* *re there target blood sugar levels for older people?*

▼
# TIP:

Y es, and you need to decide what yours are with your doctor's help. As you age, you will probably have higher targets to guard against hypoglycemia (extremely low blood sugar).

Here's a chart of ideal blood glucose target ranges. The blood glucose monitors and strips you use give either plasma or whole blood results. It is important to know which result your meter gives. Plasma results are 10–15% higher than whole blood results. These are plasma values in milligrams per deciliter (mg/dl).

| Plasma values (mg/dl) | Non-diabetes | Goal | Action suggested |
|---|---|---|---|
| Before meals | Less than 110 | 90–130 | Less than 90 or greater than 150 |
| After meals (1–2 hours) | Less than 140 | Less than 180 | Greater than 180 |
| Bedtime | Less than 120 | 110–150 | Less than 110 or greater than 180 |

# $W$hat affects my blood glucose levels?

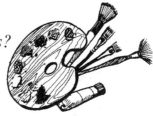

▼
## TIP:

$B$ lood glucose is never level. The ups and downs are natural and caused by several things, including:

- **Eating**. Depending on the food, glucose rises about 30 minutes after eating and will return to normal about 3 hours later. Eating large servings can raise glucose higher than you want. Lots of fat in a meal can slow the rise in blood glucose for several hours.
- **Physical activity**. Regular exercise usually lowers glucose, which makes it a valuable part of your diabetes plan. If your glucose is above 250 mg/dl and has been for some time, exercise may cause it to rise even higher.
- **Stress**. Emotional upset can cause your glucose to be high, due to a flood of stress hormones. Worrying and anxiety do it, too.
- **Illness**. Even the slightest cold can raise blood glucose.
- **Sluggish stomach function**. Sometimes food stays undigested in the stomach and is absorbed over many hours. Glucose may be up and down when you don't expect it.
- **Medications**. Some may influence blood glucose, causing it to be higher or lower than expected. Ask your doctor and pharmacist about this whenever you get a new prescription.

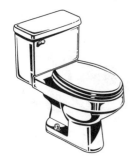

*I was recently diagnosed, and my doctor says I've probably had high blood sugar for years. What are the symptoms of high blood sugar?*

The symptoms of diabetes are complex, but the treachery is that with type 2 diabetes there may be no symptoms for many years. High blood sugar may cause symptoms such as poor healing of cuts and scratches, bacterial or yeast infections, fatigue, itching, or blurred vision. You may feel tired and cranky and refuse to get off the couch.This is true for people with type 1 or type 2 diabetes. Your symptoms came on gradually, so you didn't notice them.

If a person with type 1 diabetes forgets to take an insulin injection or doesn't take enough, his health suffers within hours or days. The body has to burn fat for fuel instead of the glucose it can't get. The symptoms of high blood sugar at these times are thirst, excessive urination, and weight loss. If your blood sugar level gets very high with type 2, you will probably have these symptoms, too.

If it is not treated, very high blood glucose can lead to severe problems.

*M*y mother lives in a nursing home. Could she get problems with very high blood glucose?

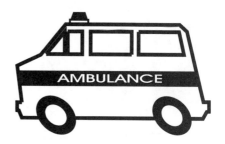

▼
## TIP:

Yes. Two serious complications can happen: ketoacidosis and hyperosmolar hyperglycemia. In both conditions:

- Dehydration is caused by high glucose, because glucose spills over into urine with great "water" loss.
- Infection is the common cause. Other causes include strokes, heart attacks, injuries, alcohol abuse, stopping or reducing insulin, and medications such as cortisone.

Ketoacidosis happens to people with type 1 diabetes. Their blood glucose is usually above 250 mg/dl. Ketoacidosis usually comes on quickly, over 24 hours, so check her ketones with urine tests every 1–4 hours until her blood glucose comes back down.

Hyperosmolar hyperglycemia happens to people with type 2 over several days to weeks. Dehydration is severe. Their blood glucose is usually above 650 mg/dl, and the patient goes into a coma, which is difficult to reverse.

Make sure the staff at the nursing home know what to watch for and what to do to prevent her from developing very high blood glucose.

 *A*<sub> </sub>*m I going to have a heart attack?*

D iabetes puts you at very high risk for a heart attack, so you should adopt the health practices of people who've already had one. This may prevent you from ever having one.

The things that contribute to developing diabetes, such as being overweight, inactivity, smoking, hypertension, and blood fat disorders, also put you at risk for heart disease. You can control these factors (lose weight, stop smoking, etc.) and reduce the added risk to your heart.

Because of the damage that diabetes does to nerve pathways, you may not be able to feel chest pain if you are having angina or a heart attack. Be aware of your blood pressure and pulse rate, especially when you are exercising. Be aware that your only symptoms of a heart attack may be tiredness, shortness of breath, or indigestion.

Ask your doctor about heart tests, such as a stress test or arteriogram. If you have heart problems, they can be treated.

# *H*ow often should I see a diabetes educator?

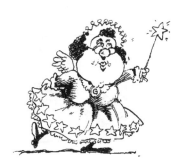

▼
## TIP:

See an educator when your diabetes is discovered to learn blood glucose monitoring, how to give insulin injections, the signs and treatment of low and high blood glucose, when to take pills, and how to be successful in lifestyle changes (such as exercise and giving up tobacco). Follow-up visits are important, too. See an educator when you have big lifestyle changes or problems with diabetes management. For example, you start exercising every day and have low blood glucose too often. An educator can help you adjust your meal plan and medication to avoid that. Or help you adjust for other health problems, or retirement. Even if everything is going smoothly, an educator can teach you the latest developments in diabetes care. Education can make you healthier.

Diabetes educators are key members of a diabetes treatment team. Chances are that you can find one in your town or a larger community nearby. Most diabetes educators are nurses or dietitians, but any health care professional with an interest in diabetes management may become trained as a certified diabetes educator (CDE).

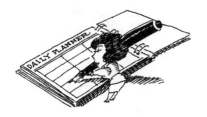

*H*ow can I organize my
diabetes care, so it doesn't
take so much time?

▼
## TIP:

**H**ere are some ideas for getting organized:

- Get diabetes education. Know what to do, why, and what to expect.
- Write things down in a daily record of blood glucose checks, food, exercise, stress, illness, or anything that affects your blood glucose. Take it with you to doctor's appointments.
- Keep your glucose monitor calibrated and in working order. Use it.
- Always carry everything you need for diabetes with you in a cooler, tote, or backpack.
- Wear a medical ID saying you have diabetes.
- Keep a list of medications, what they are for, and when you take them. Take this to your doctor's appointments.
- Learn from your experiences. Observing how your blood sugar responds to activity, medication, stress, and other things, such as eating pizza or birthday cake, helps you fine-tune your treatment plan to fit you.

*S*ince I've retired, I spend a lot of time traveling. What can I do to make sure my diabetes is under control while I'm away from home?

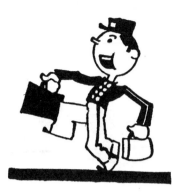

▼
## TIP:

**B**e organized! Be sure you have everything you need with you. If you're flying, make sure your medication, supplies, and extra food are in your carry-on luggage. Bring twice the amount of medications and supplies you think you need. Other things to bring are:

- A letter from your physician or health care provider stating that you have diabetes, what your insulin or medication program is, what medications are prescribed to you, and the contact phone numbers for emergencies.
- A medical ID bracelet to be worn at all times
- Enough food for 24 hours
- Copies of all your prescriptions, in case you run out while you're traveling
- Locations and phone numbers of hospitals and pharmacies in the area you will be traveling in

Keep in mind that your daily schedule will be dramatically changed while traveling. If you're traveling through different time zones, try and schedule your medication and eating regimen to your *home time zone*, not the one you're flying through. Also keep in mind that you may get more exercise than normal and be eating different foods—putting you at risk for hypoglycemia (low blood sugar).

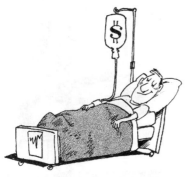

*D*iabetes is expensive, and I'm on a limited budget. Sometimes I just don't have the money to cover the cost. Are there resources available to help me out?

▼
## TIP:

Yes there are. If you have diabetes and you're on a fixed income, you're not alone in your struggle for good health and proper management. There are a variety of resources available to help you. To find out what resources are in your area, call the Eldercare Locator (funded by the Federal Administration on Aging) at 1-800-677-1116, or talk to a certified diabetes educator (CDE) (most hospitals have them on staff). Available programs vary by area, but you might find:

- special transportation arrangements to take you to your doctor
- volunteers who will stop by and see that everything's all right
- organizations that serve low-cost meals or deliver meals to your home
- free diabetes education classes and support groups
- information on special equipment that might help your needs

You may also contact your insurance company or Medicare office to see what diabetes services they cover.

*I*s the future of diabetes care bright?

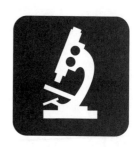

▼
# TIP:

Each year brings new therapies for diabetes. The future holds great promise with new products that will make diabetes management simpler and more effective for you. Successful islet-cell transplants are now being done. New oral medications are being developed almost yearly. Exciting progress is being made in non-injection insulin delivery systems (nasal spray and capsules). The GlucoWatch that checks glucose without requiring a drop of blood is brand new. You still need to use a regular glucose monitor to check the accuracy of the GlucoWatch, but now we have laser lancets, which are nearly painless, and the ability to take a blood sample from a forearm, which is also not painful. Dietitians are updating nutrition recommendations to make them healthy for everyone and less difficult to follow. There is research being done on how to prevent diabetes, map chromosomes (genes) and predict future health conditions, and manipulate genes to avoid or alter health conditions. The future is very bright indeed. More and more help is on the way.

# Chapter 2
# MIGHTY MEDICATIONS

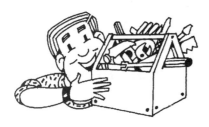

# *H*ow do pills for diabetes work?

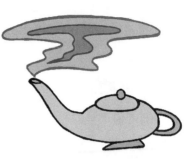

▼
## TIP:

There are several types of pills for blood glucose control in people with type 2 diabetes. They include:

- Pills that stimulate the pancreas to release insulin: sulfonylureas (such as glyburide and glipizide) and meglitinides (repaglinide [Prandin]). These medications may cause low blood glucose.
- Pills that help body cells take in glucose: thiazolidinediones (rosiglitazone and pioglitazone) and biguanides (metformin). These do not cause low blood glucose if used alone.
- Pills that block absorption of carbohydrate from the intestines: alpha-glucosidase inhibitors (such as acarbose and miglitol). These do not cause low blood glucose if used alone. Uncomfortable side effects, such as gasiness, limit the popularity of these medications.

Other types of medications are under study. Discuss your choices carefully with your health care provider, considering the cost, the number of times per day you have to take it, and side effects. Some people need to take more than one diabetes pill to control their blood glucose, and others need to move on to insulin for better control.

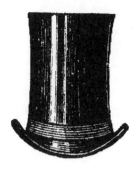

*A re there advantages to taking one diabetes pill rather than another?*

Which pill you take depends on what is causing your high blood glucose. If you need to produce more insulin, sulfonylureas and meglitinides help. Sulfonylureas have been around longest and work well, but can cause hypoglycemia and weight gain. You can't use them if you're allergic to sulfa drugs or have kidney problems. Meglitinides (Prandin) are taken before meals, so if you don't eat, you don't take it, which is handy. It's okay with kidney problems, but weight gain is possible.

Two pills increase how much glucose gets into your cells: thiazolidinediones ('glitazones) and biguanides (metformin). You take glitazones only once a day, and they lower triglyceride levels. But they cause weight gain. Metformin does not cause weight gain or low blood glucose and improves blood fats. Side effects, however, are nausea and diarrhea, and you can't take it with kidney, heart, or liver problems, or if you drink alcohol excessively.

Alpha-glucosidase inhibitors block absorption of carbohydrate in your intestines, keeping glucose lower after a meal. There's no weight gain, but gas, bloating, and diarrhea are side effects. Talk with your doctor to decide which pill will work best for you.

*W*hy aren't my new diabetes pills lowering my blood glucose?

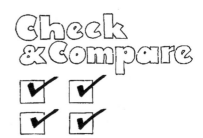

▼
## TIP:

Time is required for any new medication to start working. The time varies for the different types of pills used to treat diabetes:

- Pills that stimulate the release of insulin from the pancreas, including sulfonylureas and meglitinides, will reach full effect in one week.
- Pills that block absorption of carbohydrate from the intestinal tract work immediately and are used with each meal.
- Pills that improve the efficiency of insulin action, "insulin sensitizers," include biguanides and thiazolidinediones. Metformin (currently the only approved biguanide) reaches full effect in one week. Thiazolidinediones do not start working for approximately three weeks and may not reach full effect for ten to twelve weeks. Watch for their effect to show up on your blood glucose checks at home.

Did your doctor prescribe a thiazolidinedione (insulin sensitizer)? Take these facts into consideration when starting a new diabetes medication or when considering a change in the dose of your medication.

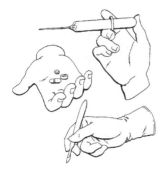

*I*t's becoming harder to control my diabetes with pills. What are the advantages and disadvantages of my taking insulin now?

▼
## TIP:

Insulin does the same thing that your body's insulin does—helps you get energy from the food you eat and thrive. As you age with type 2, the chances are you will probably need to start insulin therapy at some point. When you start is often your choice. Here are some advantages and disadvantages to using insulin:

Advantages:
- Much better blood glucose control.
- More flexibility in diabetes management. For example, you can make an on-the-spot increase in insulin dose to cover a large birthday meal, or be able to delay a meal.
- The types of insulin have different time-action patterns. Some start to work rapidly and are gone in two hours. Some act gradually over 24 hours. Pills are not so easy to adjust.

Disadvantages:
- Possibility of too low blood glucose (hypoglycemia).
- Weight gain.
- Need for injections.
- Reluctance from you or your physician.

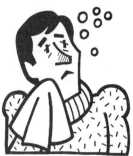

*I recently had pneumonia, and my doctor put me on insulin. Will I have to stay on insulin forever?*

No, probably not. When you're ill, your body's under a lot of stress, and this can cause your blood sugar to go a little crazy. Insulin is the best way to get things back under control. However, once you're back up to speed, you can probably return to your regular management plan.

Temporary insulin therapy may also be used when type 2 diabetes is first diagnosed, to overcome very high glucose. Once the glucose is under control, oral medication will usually do the trick.

Some people use rapid-acting insulin occasionally when they're eating a large meal, for example, at the holidays. The insulin covers the extra carbohydrate in the meal and brings their blood sugar back to normal levels after the meal.

And now for the "probably not" part. As you age, oral medications might not control your blood glucose as well as they should. To get good control and stay healthy, you might have to start using insulin. If you're to this level, you'll have to keep using insulin from then on.

*M*y doctor suggested I start using insulin. Will I be able to handle this regimen at my age?

## ▼ TIP:

You may feel scared or overwhelmed, but the mechanics of drawing the insulin dose and giving an injection are simple to do. It's learning to think like a pancreas that is the challenge. If you already have a good management plan of meal plan, exercise, and oral medications, you have experience that will help you use insulin. You will need to check your blood glucose levels more often because now they can drop too low—and you don't want that to happen. You'll need to carry snacks or glucose tablets with you at all times to bring low blood sugar back up.

You will probably start with a bedtime injection of intermediate- or long-acting insulin, such as glargine, to restore normal morning glucose so your oral medications will work better during the day. If blood glucose control worsens, you'll probably move on to several insulin injections a day. No one likes injections, but they keep you healthier. Once you face your fear and get some practice, you'll be amazed at how well you do.

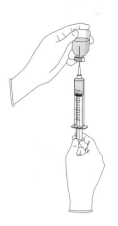

*I* *can't see well. How can I measure my*
*insulin dose?*

▼
# TIP:

S everal devices are available to help you draw up and
measure insulin when you can't see.

- Syringe magnifiers are magnifying glasses that attach to the
  insulin syringe, making the numbers larger.
- There are several non-visual insulin measurement aides.
  These devices hold the syringe and the insulin bottle. A
  predetermined "stop" on the device halts the insulin
  syringe plunger at a given dose. Or, a slide moves the
  syringe plunger with a "click" sound that indicates each
  unit of insulin drawn into the syringe.
- Needle guides hold syringe and insulin bottle in place for
  syringe filling or have a funnel shape that fits over the
  insulin bottle and directs the syringe needle tip to the
  insulin bottle stopper.
- Insulin pens have an insulin reservoir, a double-ended
  needle (one end in the insulin reservoir, the other for you),
  and a dose-dialing mechanism. You can set the dose
  visually or by counting off the clicks. Two styles of such
  pens are available—disposable and refillable.

Ask your diabetes educator or occupational therapist for
suggestions and help learning how to use them.

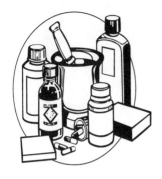

*I take a lot of non-diabetes medications. Can any of these affect my blood glucose?*

## ▼
## TIP:

If you take a sulfonylurea or Prandin, your glucose may go too low if you are also taking:

- Nonsteroidal anti-inflammatory medications, such as aspirin or ibuprofen
- Sulfa drugs and certain antibiotics
- Monoamine oxidase inhibitors (MAOs) (for depression)
- Beta-blockers (for heart problems or high blood pressure)

Anyone's blood glucose may be made higher by:

- Cold remedies, such as ephedrine or pseudoephedrine
- Phenothiazines (for nausea and anxiety)
- Phenytoin (for peripheral neuropathy or seizures)
- Diuretics (to remove fluid from the body)
- Corticosteroids, such as cortisone or prednisone
- Thyroid medications
- Estrogen medications
- Calcium channel blockers (not recommended for people with diabetes)
- Nicotinic acid (for abnormal blood fats)

Ask your doctor or pharmacist how your medications will affect your blood glucose and be alert to your own reactions to a new drug.

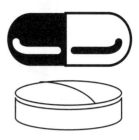

*I*'m retired and on a tight budget. Can I cut my diabetes pills in half?

▼
## TIP:

If you're a thrifty medical consumer, you've probably thought of buying pills containing larger doses of medication, and then just using the portion you need, so you can save money on prescription prices. However, there are some things you should know.

If you just break the pill, the pieces may not contain the same amount of medication and may not work the same way. Pills that are "scored"—meaning they have a line cut into them—and that *do not* have a special coating may be broken along the line, and both halves will have the same amount of medication. However, a shiny tablet without a line in it or a capsule might not work correctly if you break it in two. The coating on the pill may be necessary to control how fast or where the pill is absorbed in your body.

Leave shiny, un-scored pills as they are, unless you ask your pharmacist if it is okay to break the pills into pieces.

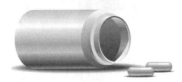 *I've heard that taking an aspirin everyday is recommended for seniors. Is this true if I have diabetes?*

# ▼
# TIP:

Probably. As the years go by, everyone runs a higher risk of heart attack, stroke, and poor circulation, whether they have diabetes or not. This higher risk is caused by atherosclerosis, or hardening of the arteries. This condition is made even worse by thromboxane, a chemical in your blood. Aspirin helps by blocking the production of thromboxane. So, aspirin is especially helpful for you with diabetes because you have an even higher risk for heart attack and stroke.

As you and your physician decide whether you should take a daily aspirin, consider the following:

- The low dose treatment is 81–325 mg of enteric-coated aspirin per day. This is lower than the amount you take for aches and pains, but it gives you the benefits without many of the side effects.
- People with aspirin allergy, bleeding tendencies, recent bleeding in the stomach or intestinal tract, anticoagulant therapy, and liver troubles should not use aspirin.
- Low dose aspirin will not trigger or irritate diabetes-related eye problems.

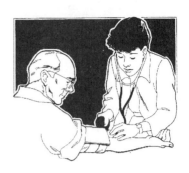

*I've developed high blood
pressure. What types of pills are
available to control it, and how will
they affect my diabetes?*

▼
## TIP:

There are five types of blood pressure medication. They may be started in any order and added if one or more do not get the job done. Each has advantages and disadvantages:

**Thiazide diuretics** are also useful in controlling fluid retention. Side effects include blood fat (lipid) abnormalities, mild elevation in blood glucose, possible low potassium, and elevation in uric acid (linked to gout).

**Beta-blockers** are also beneficial in reducing recurring heart problems after a heart attack. Side effects include lipid abnormalities, masking of the symptoms of low blood glucose, cool hands and feet, and making asthma worse.

**Angiotensin-converting enzyme (ACE) inhibitors** are also proven to reduce or protect against diabetes-related kidney problems. Side effects include raising potassium levels and reducing kidney function. Cough may be a side effect (a newer medication is less likely to cause cough).

**Calcium antagonists** do not affect lipids or blood glucose. Side effects include fluid retention (swelling of the feet) and constipation.

**Alpha-1-receptor blockers** benefit lipid levels and improve insulin sensitivity. A possible serious side effect is low blood pressure when standing, causing dizziness.

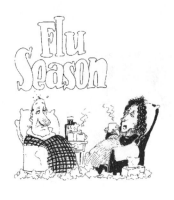

*Do I need flu and pneumonia shots?*

▼
## TIP:

Whether to have influenza and pneumonia immunizations is a personal decision. However, people over the age of 64 will usually benefit from the protection conferred by these injections. If flu or pneumonia are "in the air", immunizations will prevent the illnesses or make them less severe.

Getting a flu shot is strongly recommended in September of each year. The vaccine should not be used if you are allergic to chicken eggs (the vaccine is prepared in a chicken egg environment) or to other components of the vaccine, or in people with a past history of Guillain-Barré syndrome (a rare nerve disorder occasionally linked to immunizations).

The pneumonia vaccine protects against a relatively common type—pneumococcal pneumonia. A one-time dose of vaccine is recommended for people over the age of 64. If you got a dose before age 65, a one-time re-vaccination is recommended. Almost half of the people receiving this injection will have flu-like side effects lasting up to two days.

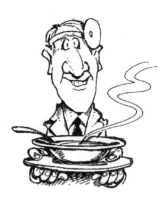

*A* *re there vitamins or minerals I*
*should be taking to help with the*
*aging process?*

▼

## TIP:

If you follow a meal plan with fresh vegetables, fruit, lean meats and fish, eggs, and whole grains, there's no need for supplemental vitamins. You also need healthy fats like olive oil in your diet. Most people don't eat this well, however. Talk with your doctor or dietitian about taking vitamins or using herbal supplements. Be honest because these can interact with your other medications. Some herbs, like Siberian ginseng, have had years of research done on their benefits for older people, but most have not.

You may need a calcium supplement to keep bones strong. There are also special situations where you may need supplements:

- If you are being fed through an IV tube, you may need chromium.
- Magnesium deficiency can cause insulin resistance, high blood pressure, and high blood glucose, but deficiency is not common. Unless you have low blood levels of magnesium, don't worry about a supplement.
- If you are taking diuretics, you might need potassium. But, you may need to restrict it if it is too high from kidney problems or from taking ACE inhibitors for high blood pressure.

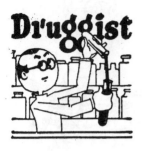

**Druggist**

*I take so many medications that it's hard for me to keep them straight. What can I do?*

▼
## TIP:

O rganize your medications to avoid mixing medicines, taking the wrong medications, or not taking the medicine at all. Try these tips:

- Get a plastic pill organizer with as many sections as you need to keep track of what you're taking and when you're taking it. Refill it at the same time each week.
- Keep an updated list of all your medications with you at all times.
- Tell your doctor every medication you take (including herbs, vitamins, and over-the-counter medications).
- Try to have all your prescriptions filled at the same pharmacy.
- Make sure you understand the instructions and dosages. If you can't read the label, have someone read it for you.
- Mark off each medication as you take it on a calendar.
- Label the caps of your pills with big letters, so you can see which is which. For example, a big, yellow "BP" for blood pressure pills.
- Put bright stickers or tape on each bottle, so you can tell them apart.
- Be aware that some diabetes pills look like artificial sweeteners—don't confuse them. One woman put three in her husband's oatmeal, causing very low blood sugar!

*I*'ve recently had an amputation and doing day-to-day activities is a big challenge. What can I do?

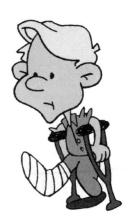

▼
## TIP:

Ask your doctor for a referral to an occupational therapist. In fact, anyone who has trouble with daily activities for any reason whatsoever (such as arthritis or poor vision), probably should see an occupational therapist for help. Don't let the name fool you. An occupational therapist isn't someone who just helps you with challenges at your job. The therapist provides you with physical therapy to increase your strength and mobility and training—often in your home—in better ways to deal with a variety of physical ailments. He or she can show you the nifty inventions that can help you and how to use them. If you've had an amputation, you'll need to learn to do things differently and safely to prevent further injury to that leg and to the rest of you, too! You may need to learn to use a cane or a wheelchair, need grab bars to get onto the toilet, and into and out of the bathtub. The therapist can do a survey of your home and suggest adjustments that will make things easier for you.

# Chapter 3
# FOOD, GLORIOUS FOOD

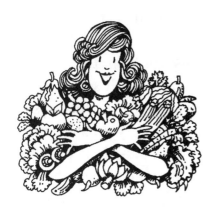

*H*<sup></sup>*ow can I eat healthy?*

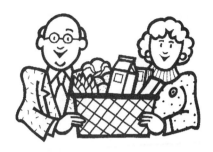

▼
## TIP:

Ask your doctor to refer you to a registered dietitian (RD) who can design a meal plan for your food likes and dislikes and your cooking ability. Try these tips:

- Eat more fresh (or frozen) vegetables and fruit daily.
- Eat more greens, like romaine, watercress, spinach, and arugula every day
- Drink 6–8 glasses of water a day.
- Eat breakfast (try oatmeal).
- Eat an egg. It's a perfect food.
- Use olive oil to cook and add nuts to your oatmeal—for healthy fat.
- Stop eating processed foods. (Read the ingredients— partially hydrogenated oil is an unhealthy fat).
- Measure your servings with a measuring cup or food scale.
- Try 5 or 6 small meals a day.
- Use herbs and spices instead of salt and fat.
- Buy a healthy cookbook.
- Stop smoking to improve your sense of taste and smell.
- Think about the energy the food brings you and what you intend to do with the energy. Participate in the dance of life.

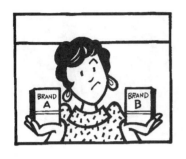

$W$*hy would I learn to "count carbs"?*

It is the carbohydrate in food that raises your blood glucose. If you count how much carbohydrate (carb) is in your meal, you'll know how much to eat. Carbohydrate is in grains, beans, fruits, milk, and sweets. You can look up how much carbohydrate is in a serving of food on food labels and in "carb count" books. Make sure the serving you eat is the same size as the one on the label or in the book. Add up the carb in your meal and write it in your record. Check your blood glucose two hours later and record that, too. After a week or two you'll see how high certain amounts of carb raise your blood sugar. If you try to eat about the same amount of carb at the same times each day, you may get better diabetes control.

Carb raises blood glucose. Exercise and diabetes medication lower it. If you exercise after eating, record that. If you are going to eat more carb than usual—at a birthday party for example—then you know you need to take a walk afterwards or adjust your diabetes medication to bring the blood glucose level back down. You can adjust insulin to the carb you eat and some of the diabetes pills. Ask your doctor or diabetes educator for help with this.

*F*or years I've heard that people with diabetes can't eat sugar. Is this true?

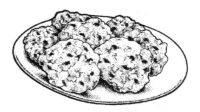

▼
# TIP:

No, it's not true. Twenty years of research have shown that sugar is just another carbohydrate. As far as your blood glucose is concerned, a brownie and a baked potato have about the same effect.

It is the carbohydrate in foods that raises blood glucose. Carbohydrate—whether in grains, beans, fruit, milk, or sweets—turns into glucose and is used for fuel. So, carbohydrates like potatoes and bread raise blood glucose the same way that table sugar (another carbohydrate) does. Don't focus on the sugar; focus on the total amount of carbohydrate in the meal.

Table sugar is considered a "bad guy" because it gives you calories but no vitamins or minerals—these are empty calories. If you want a natural sugar that is packaged with vitamins and minerals, you can choose a piece of fresh fruit! But if you want to eat dessert, go ahead and try just 2 or 3 bites. You can trade the carb in the bites of brownie for a piece of bread or serving of rice in your meal plan.

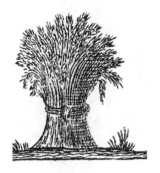

# *W*hy should I eat more fiber?

▼
## TIP:

Fiber makes your body work better. It improves your digestion and prevents constipation. It is found in whole grains,
beans, fruits, and vegetables. It's on the food label, too. Try to
eat 20–35 grams of fiber a day. There are two types of fiber:

- Insoluble fiber is in whole grain cereals and breads. It grabs
  onto liquid as it travels your gastrointestinal tract. That's
  good because the combination of fiber and liquid pushes
  food through more quickly. Insoluble fiber promotes a
  bulkier and softer bowel movement and gives you other
  health benefits—preventing hemorrhoids, diverticulosis,
  and colon and rectal cancer.
- Soluble fiber is in beans, peas, oats, and barley. It can prevent your body from absorbing cholesterol and glucose.
  But to lower your blood cholesterol or glucose with it, you
  would have to eat a very large amount.

If you count carbs and there are more than 5 grams of fiber
in the serving you eat, subtract the number of grams of fiber
from the grams of total carbohydrate. Use that number for the
carb count in the food. The carb from fiber will not raise your
blood glucose.

*101 Tips for Aging Well with Diabetes*

*W*hy do I have to drink 6–8 glasses of water a day?

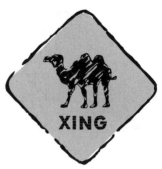

XING

▼
## TIP:

W ater is vital to every process and system in your body. It keeps you healthy. When blood sugars run high, you're at risk of getting dehydrated because your body tries to flush out the extra glucose in your blood through urination. The flushed-out fluids need to be replaced. If they're not, you get sick.

Be sure to drink water throughout the day. Why not get a measuring cup and check the amount of water that your favorite drinking glass or water bottle will hold? You can make this the week you add more water to your routine.

Coffee and tea with caffeine and carbonated sodas are diuretics and can remove water from your system. Drinking plain water is the best way to get the fluid you need.

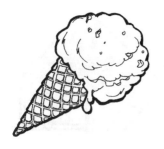

# $W$$hy$ is fat in food so bad?

▼
## TIP:

$F$ats are not the root of all evil. In fact, fats:

- help your body and brain work
- transport essential vitamins (A, D, and E)
- make skin and hair look healthy
- reduce hunger feelings
- make food taste good

It's just that too much of a good thing is bad. Excessive amounts of fat in your diet are linked to a variety of health issues. This is especially true as you age. Excessive amounts of fat in your bloodstream can stick to your arteries causing them to become smaller. When you have diabetes, these fats become stickier and cause even more buildup. As you age, you get more and more buildup, narrowing your arteries, too. When the space inside your arteries shrinks, you develop high blood pressure (hypertension), and a higher risk for heart attack and stroke.

When you eat wisely, choosing healthier fats such as olive oil instead of butter or margarine (or even dark chocolate instead of milk chocolate), and cut some processed or fried foods out of your meal plan, you're seriously reducing the risks to your health.

# *H*ow much fat should I have in my diet?

**Y**ou need a little fat every day—but only a little because fat has so many calories. One gram of fat has 9 calories. If you read food labels, you'll see the calories from fat add up quickly. Fat should only make up about 30% of the total calories you eat in a day (if you eat 2000 calories a day, then 600 of those can come from fat).

There are actually three types of fat in the food you eat—monounsaturated, polyunsaturated, and saturated fats. The healthiest are monounsaturated, found in olive oil and nuts. Polyunsaturated are the next healthiest (found in canola and corn oils). Saturated fats in meat and dairy products are the least healthy.

If your blood fat levels are too high, you may need to eat different amounts of the fats, and you might need prescription medication. If you need to lose weight, pay attention to how much fat you eat because fat has more calories than protein or carbohydrate. Get the help of an RD who can help you make a meal plan with healthy amounts of the three kinds of fat.

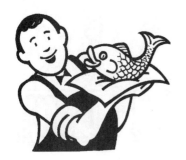

*I'm confused about fats. Which ones can I eat?*

▼

## TIP:

The healthiest fats are found in olives, olive oil, and canola oil. The fats in nuts, seeds, and avocados help protect your heart and improve your health. Butter is okay in small amounts for taste! Eat whole grains and legumes like soy.

Probably the worst fat is trans fat. It is in most processed foods, such as crackers and cookies. Look for it on the list of ingredients as partially hydrogenated oil. Liquid oil is treated with hydrogen to make it solid at room temperature. Hydrogenation makes a liquid fat—which is usually healthier—into a saturated fat, which takes away the health benefit, as with margarine. Foods that are fried in most restaurants also have trans fats, which is why you choose a baked potato instead of French fries. If you want fries, fry them at home and discard the oil afterward or make oven-fried potatoes with less oil.

Research is showing that eliminating trans fats from your diet dramatically improves your health by lowering your risk of cancer and heart disease.

# Chapter 4
# EVERY BODY IS BEAUTIFUL

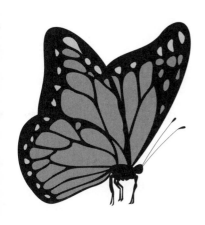

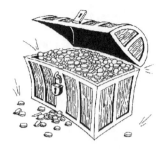

*W*hat does exercise do for me?

▼
# TIP:

The benefits of exercise are many, and they include:

- Strong muscles
- More energy
- One-pound weight loss for every 3,500 calories burned
- Improved mobility and range of joint motion
- Enhanced quality of life and independence
- A better mental attitude and self-image
- Improved blood glucose control
- Reduced chance of heart attacks and strokes
- Improved cholesterol and lipids
- Improved blood pressure
- Improved blood flow (reduced chances of conditions such as phlebitis)
- Improved appetite
- Improved enjoyment of sex
- Improved ability to play with your grandchildren
- Respect from your children

Exercise keeps you young and healthy. Are there any good reasons not to exercise?

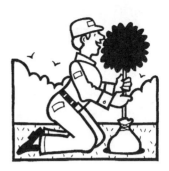

*I*'m not the young pup I used to be. What kinds of exercise are best for me?

▼
## TIP:

The best exercise is one you will do regularly. Aerobic exercise (exercise that raises the heart rate and feels like work) is best, but just about any physical activity is a step in the right direction.

There are three basic approaches to exercise and all are beneficial:

- **Lifestyle approach.** Stand rather than sit. Take the stairs. Lift everyday weights (groceries, bottles of water, bags of flour). Garden. Bend and stretch.
- **Non-competitive activity.** Compete against the clock rather than other athletes. Organize a walking group. Take a yoga class. Lift weights. Swim. Bicycle.
- **Competitive sports.** Just that. Everything from golf to running a marathon.

Exercise regularly, three to four times a week. Aerobic sessions can be 20–60 minutes, but start with 5 minutes if you've never exercised. Mix up your workouts with yoga twice a week and lift light weights once or twice a week, too. Ease your way into it. The benefits are many. For example, yoga increases your flexibility, strength, coordination, and balance, and it reduces stress. It can lower blood glucose levels, too.

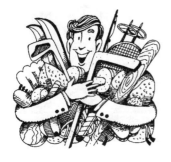

# $W$*hy do I need to burn more calories?*

▼
## TIP:

$B$urning calories is how you lose weight. You lose one pound for every 3,500 calories you burn and don't replace with more calories. The table shows the calories burned by a 150-pound person doing 30 minutes of each of the activities.

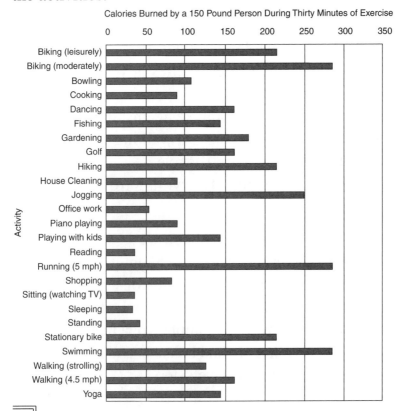

Calories Burned by a 150 Pound Person During Thirty Minutes of Exercise

*T*his year I'll be celebrating my 75th birthday. Am I too old to exercise?

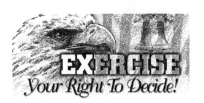

▼
## TIP:

**T**he answer to that question is always going to be "no." You're never too old to exercise. The benefits you receive with regular exercise are always there. Start walking, swimming, gardening, or doing something you enjoy now, and you'll benefit every system in your body and reduce all your health risks. You won't get frail, and you won't have to depend on others to do things for you. Now that's a birthday present!

Recent studies have shown that strength training in 90-year-olds produces muscle mass just as it does in 20-year-olds. Now, this doesn't mean you'll be winning bodybuilding competitions—even though we know of an 83-year-old lady who is—but it does mean that you can get benefits from strength training no matter how old you are. Weight lifting—even 1-lb weights—increases muscle and bone, which keeps you stronger and gives you endurance. And muscle burns calories even at rest—keeping weight and blood glucose levels in control.

So grumble if you will, but do it. Strong muscles mean improved health, well-being, and longevity.

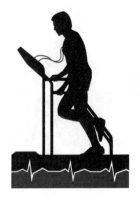

*H*ow do I know that I'm healthy enough to exercise?

▼
## TIP:

**B**efore starting an exercise program, you should have a health evaluation, especially if you:

- Are over 35 years old
- Have had type 2 diabetes for more than 10 years or type 1 diabetes for more than 15 years
- Have diabetes-related eye or kidney problems (retinopathy or nephropathy)
- Have poor circulation in your legs
- Have neuropathy preventing an increase in heart rate with exercise
- Have high blood pressure
- Smoke

Your doctor can help you determine whether you have any conditions that would limit the way you exercise. If you have eye problems, don't do jumping or jarring exercise or lift heavy weights. If you have lost feeling in your feet, be careful not to injure your feet, and you may find swimming preferable to jogging. An exercise tolerance test is important if you have heart disease.

Exercise will improve your diabetes control, your blood pressure, and your circulation.

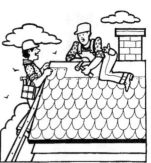

*I take insulin. Do I need to take special precautions when I exercise?*

▼
## TIP:

If you take insulin, sulfonylureas, or meglitinide (Prandin), you need to watch that your blood sugar does not drop too low during and for hours after exercise. If the exercise is unusual, vigorous, or long-lasting, you may need to check your blood sugar during it and after. Have plenty of snacks to eat. In general:

- If your glucose levels are below 100 mg/dl, you need to eat 15–30 grams of carbohydrate.
- Always have carbohydrate food close at hand. You can carry glucose gel or tablets, peanut butter crackers, or a bike bottle filled with fruit juice.
- You may be surprised by lower than usual blood glucose levels during the night or the next day! You need to adjust your diabetes treatment for this.
- Avoid exercise if your blood glucose level is above 240 mg/dl and ketones are present in your urine, or if blood glucose is above 300 mg/dl without ketones in the urine. Under these conditions, exercise may actually raise your blood glucose.

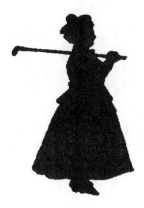

*I*'ve had type 2 diabetes for 20 years and want to start exercising. What do I need to know?

▼
## TIP:

S tart slowly with walking or a yoga or tai chi class. Begin like this:

- Before any physical activity, warm up your bones, joints, and muscles for 5–10 minutes, by swinging your arms and marching, for example.
- After you are warmed-up, gently stretch for another 5–10 minutes. Never stretch cold muscles. Don't bounce.
- After exercise, spend 5–10 minutes cooling down—moving slower and slower. Try some yoga stretches.
- You need to move quickly enough to get your heart and lungs working.
- Protect your feet. Wear good walking or running shoes with cushioned innersoles that fit well. Wear socks made of a fabric that keeps your feet dry.
- Inspect your feet regularly for blisters or injury.
- Drink water before, during, and after exercise.
- Lift some light weights. Even 1-lb cans of soup can build muscle—and muscle burns calories even when you are at rest! Don't carry weights while you're walking because that can damage your wrist, elbow, and shoulder joints. Never wear ankle weights while walking!
- Keep your knees slightly bent, not locked.

*I* *have arthritis and neuropathy*
*in my feet and legs. How can I*
*exercise?*

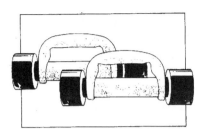

▼
**TIP:**

Where there's a will, there's a way. Swimming is good, but you need weight-bearing exercise to protect your bones. You might try yoga or tai-chi for no-impact exercise. You can lift weights and do yoga stretches sitting in a chair or on the floor. Wave two long scarves up, down, and around while listening to music to increase the range of motion in your arms and shoulders and get your heart rate going. Write the alphabet in the air with your pointed toes. There are exercise books and videotapes especially for people who have to exercise sitting down. If you start looking for ways to accomplish your goal, you will find them.

If you have other complications, such as retinopathy or high blood pressure, don't lift heavy weights or bend way over with your head hanging down.

After exercise, massage your knees with peanut or olive oil. Arnica oil (found at health food stores) is good for muscle and bone aches, too. Make sure you are getting enough calcium and magnesium in meals or supplements. Be sure to check your feet for redness, bruises, or blisters every time you exercise.

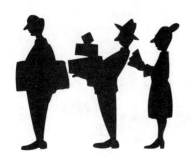

*F*rom middle age on, what is a realistic weight goal?

This is a hard question to answer because no two bodies are built exactly the same. Your body type is strongly influenced by the genes passed down from your folks, and if you have a large body type, you're always going to be bigger. Just because you weigh more or less than other people your same height, does not mean that you're over- or underweight. People are just built differently.

Don't take models or movie stars as a proper gauge. The average woman in the United States is 5'4" and weighs 152 pounds. The best way to gauge your ideal weight is to recall what you weighed at age 18–20 and add another 20 pounds "for the years." This, of course, is not completely accurate, since what you weighed at age 19 may not have been an ideal weight (especially now, as obesity among young people rises) and 20 extra pounds might be a little generous on a small body frame. But this is a pretty good working number.

To be more accurate about your ideal weight, talk with your physician. For most people, losing 20 pounds will improve their blood glucose numbers.

*D* oes diabetes have an impact on osteoporosis in men and women?

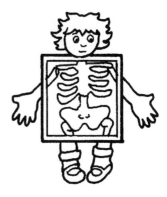

## ▼ TIP:

**P** eople with diabetes tend to have a higher rate of osteoporosis, so taking steps to prevent it would be worth your while. Osteoporosis is a loss of bone mass causing the bones to weaken and eventually break.

Osteoporosis is caused by many things, including:

- not doing enough weight-bearing exercise
- not getting enough calcium (1,000–1,500 mg) and vitamin D (800 IU) daily
- reduced levels of estrogen or testosterone, as happens later in life
- an overactive thyroid
- using certain medications such as cortisone
- smoking
- drinking too much alcohol

There are medical tests to measure bone mass and see whether you have osteoporosis. You may want to include more calcium in your meal plan or take a supplement. You can lift light weights and benefit your bones. Walking is good. Women's bones may be helped by estrogen therapy at menopause, and men's by testosterone therapy.

# Chapter 5
# WHAT'S COMMON,
# WHAT'S NOT

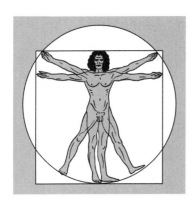

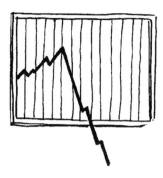

*H*ow do I recognize low blood
glucose, and how do I treat it?

▼
## TIP:

*W*hen glucose drops below 60–70 mg/dl, you will probably have symptoms, such as anxiety, sweating,
headache, hunger, numbness, heart pounding, shakiness, or
weakness. Learn what your symptoms are.

You must eat or drink carbohydrate as soon as you get the
warning signs! If you ignore them, your glucose may fall
below 30–40 mg/dl, and you may fall into a coma. To treat
low blood glucose:

■ Eat or drink food or liquid containing 15 grams of carbohydrate. Examples are 4 oz fruit juice or regular (not diet) soft
   drink, 3 graham crackers, 4 teaspoons sugar, or
   1 tablespoon honey.
■ Wait 15–20 minutes and check your blood glucose. If it's
   still below 70 mg/dl, eat 15 grams of carb and check it
   again in 15–20 minutes.
■ Repeat until your blood glucose is above 70 mg/dl.
■ If the next meal is more than an hour away, eat some
   cheese and crackers or half a meat sandwich (protein and
   carb) to keep your glucose level up.
■ Do not eat or drink too much carbohydrate. You don't want
   your glucose level to go too high.

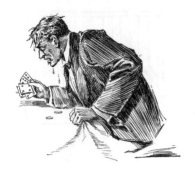

*I*s hypoglycemia (low blood sugar) more dangerous in seniors?

Yes, severely low blood sugar can cause you to pass out and fall down. For 12-year-olds, that's not too bad. When their blood sugar rises, they hop up and move on. For you, however, falling down can break bones. The danger of breaking a hip or leg is much greater as we age. And the injury may not heal properly. There is also danger with passing out when you're driving a car, mowing the lawn, or operating any kind of machinery.

If you're older, hypoglycemia can also cause a stroke. You want to do whatever you can to avoid hypoglycemia. Check your blood sugar, don't guess what it is. Eat on schedule, and if you get exercise, eat a snack. Keep a carbohydrate food, such as a juice box, with you all the time. You might want to keep your blood sugar level slightly higher than the suggested levels for younger people. Talk with your doctor about the best target levels for you and about how to adjust your diabetes care plan to reach them.

*D*oes my risk for complications increase with age?

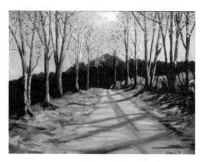

The longer that you have high blood glucose levels, the higher your risk for developing complications from diabetes. In some ways, that means it doesn't matter how old you are or even how long you've had diabetes. What does matter is how long your diabetes has been out of control and how far out of control it has been. A 50-year-old man who has let his blood glucose run high for 10 years may be at a greater risk for diabetes-related complications than an 80-year-old woman who has controlled her glucose well for more than 30 years. As a rule, however, the older you get, the more at risk you are for developing complications.

The good news is that the better you control your blood glucose, the smaller your risks for serious complications. Every bit of improvement in blood glucose control will yield benefits in long-term health and well being. It's worth the time and the effort to do it!

*M*y vision fluctuates between blurry and clear. My eyesight hasn't been good for a long time, but it's never done this. Is this retinopathy?

▼
## TIP:

If your vision improves on its own, it's not permanent damage or retinopathy. This does indicate, however, that your diabetes is out of control. The changes in your vision are due to wild swings in blood glucose, which then trigger ebb and flow of fluid in the eyes. When the level of glucose in your blood increases, the body requires more fluid to maintain a healthy balance elsewhere. Some fluid can come from your eyes, which will affect the function and structure of the eye. Blurred vision results.

The cure? Focus on diabetes control. Postpone an eye exam until you've brought some order to your blood sugar levels, which can take several weeks. Don't buy new glasses every time your vision changes because the shifting blood sugar will keep changing the way your eyes work. Spend some time on planning your meals and getting some exercise to bring your blood glucose levels nearer normal. This symptom is just another way that your body shows you when your system is out of balance.

Get a dilated eye exam every year to check for retinopathy.

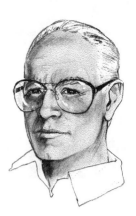

*I* *cannot see well anymore and thought it was because I was getting older. Could this be caused by diabetes?*

▼
## TIP:

Yes, over time, high levels of blood glucose can injure blood vessels in your retina, the "screen" on the back of your eye that sends images to the brain. The damage is called retinopathy, and it's common. Many new blood vessels grow on the retina and some break, leaking blood that obscures vision and scarring the retina, which affects your vision, too.

In early stages, the only symptom may be blurred vision or no symptoms at all. This is why it's so important to have yearly dilated eye exams with an ophthalmologist. Your ophthalmologist can detect retinopathy early and begin treatment, which is how you save your eyesight. Laser surgery may be required, and it is effective, so don't be afraid to try it.

Like all diabetes-related complications, the best way to treat and prevent retinopathy is to control blood sugar. By managing it and getting regular eye examinations, you can drastically reduce any chances of serious vision problems.

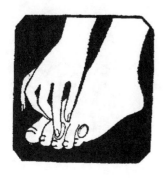

*I have heard horror stories about diabetes and amputations. What can diabetes do to my feet?*

▼
## TIP:

Diabetes can put you at risk for serious injury to your feet for several reasons.

- **Peripheral neuropathy** (nerve damage) causes numbness, burning, tingling, weakness, and decreased sweating. The numbness is perhaps most important, because you can't feel pain or changes in temperature. This is why a person can walk around with a nail poking through his shoe and not know it, or burn her feet on hot sand at the beach. You have to learn to "feel" for your numb feet. Never go barefoot, and always look inside your shoes for nails or foreign objects.

- **Bone and joint deformities** (bunions, arthritic bumps, or toes that turn downward) rub against shoes and pressure points develop. These can wear through the skin, causing foot ulcers. Make sure your shoes fit, and see a doctor immediately if you get a sore on your foot. Don't wait until it's infected.

- **Reduced blood circulation** interferes with healing of foot ulcers. White blood cells and antibiotics that fight infection can't get where they need to go.

- **Infection** is more likely to happen in the dry, cracked skin that diabetes can cause. Keep your feet clean and dry and apply a good moisturizing cream every day (but not between your toes).

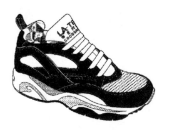

*A*m I going to have to have my *foot amputated?*

Not if you take care of yourself. Learn to think for your feet. You can:

- Never go barefoot, not even in your house.
- Have your feet checked at least once a year by your doctor. Get a "monofilament" test for loss of feeling.
- Check your feet daily. Use a mirror to see the bottoms of your feet. Run your hands over them to feel any changes.
- Wash your feet daily in warm soapy water and dry them thoroughly.
- Check inside your shoes before you put them on for nails, rips, and foreign objects.
- Only wear shoes and socks that fit. Our feet get larger as we age, so don't wear old shoes you've saved for special occasions.
- Trim toenails carefully. Get help from a podiatrist if you cannot see well or you've lost feeling in your feet.
- Avoid burns from hot water, sand, or pavement.
- Don't do bathroom surgery on your feet. Let the doctor do it.
- If you get a callus, find out what's causing it. Have your feet changed shape, so your shoes don't fit? Do you need to see a specialist to evaluate the changes in the shape of your feet?

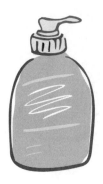

*I*s it safe for me to use creams and lotions on my feet?

When buying over-the-counter products, keep these points in mind:

- Dry skin benefits from moisturizing creams. Apply it daily after your bath or shower to prevent skin cracks and infection that may creep in through such cracks. Cost doesn't show how good the cream is—start low. You can use olive or peanut oil and wear socks to bed.
- Do not confuse dry skin with skin infection—let your doctor see it. Infections require special therapy, but some, such as athlete's foot, can be treated with over-the-counter medicines. Just make sure your physician approves of your choice. If there is redness, heat, or swelling anywhere on your feet, see your doctor immediately.
- Do not cut on corns and calluses. Better to soften them with moisturizing lotion and file them down with an Emory board. Find out what's causing the callus—a change in foot shape? A poorly fitting shoe?
- Never use over-the-counter products to remove corns or calluses! Many contain acid, which burns away tissue, causing inflammation, and that may lead to infection.

*M*y feet hurt, and I think I'm developing neuropathy. What can I expect and how can I treat the symptoms?

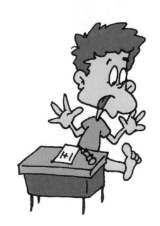

▼
## TIP:

What you can expect is discomfort—discomfort in your feet, hands, or perhaps throughout your body. Unfortunately, this is the hardest part of neuropathy to treat. There are many medications available to help keep the pain under control, from antidepressants to capsaicin cream made from hot peppers. Physical therapy to stretch sore muscles may also be useful. However, pain therapy is most successful when supervised by a physician educated in pain management. The nerve damage may progress to the point of numbness in your feet and legs. This is when you must take great care to protect your feet from any injury and to wear shoes and socks that fit well.

You may develop muscle weakness, for example, weakness in your lower leg that results in foot drop and a slapping gait when you walk. This can be managed by using a thin, right-angled support that runs down the back of your lower leg and into your shoes to support the bottom of your foot.

The best way to prevent and, in some cases, to heal neuropathy is to control your diabetes.

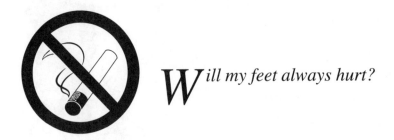

*W*ill *my feet always hurt?*

No, they won't. If you catch neuropathy early, you have a chance to reverse the effects it has on your body. Getting your blood glucose under control before the condition advances and your feet get completely numb is the first—and biggest—step. The next step is to control factors that are linked to the development of neuropathy. These include:

- High blood fats levels
- High blood pressure
- Smoking
- Excessive alcohol consumption
- Uncontrolled diabetes

Now, you need to know that as you improve your diabetes control, pain in your feet and hands may get worse. Hang in there—this is temporary. The important thing to remember is that the earlier you start to treat the condition, the better. Once your feet have gone numb, chances are you won't get the feeling back. Don't let neuropathy get out of hand. Fight back early!

*W*hat is neuropathy?

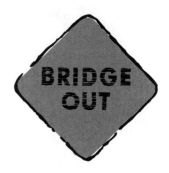

BRIDGE
OUT

**P**lain and simple, it's pretty scary stuff. Neuropathy is a long-term complication of diabetes, which results in nerve damage. Unfortunately, the signs are often overlooked, leaving you with a bad condition that just gets worse. When your doctor starts rattling off four syllable words, check these definitions to know what he's talking about.

- **Distal symmetrical polyneuropathy** involves your feet and hands, most often the feet. Symptoms usually involve discomfort (pins and needles, burning, or no feeling at all) or weakness.
- **Autonomic neuropathy** affects the part of the nervous system we don't control consciously, such as the nerves that regulate blood pressure, sweating, digestion, and bladder function.
- **Entrapment neuropathy** is caused by a squeezing of the nerves, as in carpal tunnel syndrome.

The way to avoid developing neuropathy or to improve it is to get your blood glucose levels nearer your target goals.

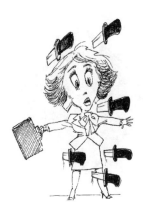

# W*hat is causing my leg pain?*

▼
## TIP:

Poor circulation could cause it, and walking can improve it. If your leg hurts, stop walking while the pain eases, and then walk a bit more. Your persistence causes your body to form new pathways for the blood to circulate.

In his late 50s, Ed has had diabetes for 20 years. Retinopathy and peripheral neuropathy handicap his running skills but do not diminish his enthusiasm or discipline. He is out there, a tube of glucose gel stuck in his headband, exercising regularly, doing races every month. He is fit and healthy to his limits.

In recent weeks, however, Ed has developed pain after exercise in his right calf and is not able to maintain his exercise schedule. He is worried that diabetes has caused poor circulation. Examination revealed nothing more than a pulled calf muscle. A brief course of physical therapy restored Ed's muscle, and he is back on the running circuit.

The moral? People with diabetes may be at risk for diabetes-related conditions. However, they are people who just happen to have diabetes. They are also entitled to have the common ailments that happen to everyone in the human race. Don't blame everything on your diabetes.

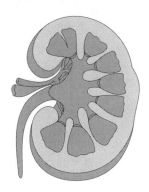

*A*<sup>*m I going to lose my kidneys?*</sup>

# TIP:

Not necessarily. You can do things to protect them. People with diabetes tend to overwork their kidneys when they have high blood glucose—the kidneys have to flush out the excess sugar—so uncontrolled diabetes can lead to kidney problems. Injury to your delicate kidney structures and tiny blood vessels may cause the filters to leak, which allows albumin (a protein) to pass into your urine. A small amount of leaking albumin is called microalbuminuria. This is the beginning of nephropathy.

If the overworking of your kidneys continues unchecked for a number of years, larger amounts of albumin are released into your urine. High blood pressure usually develops. Your kidneys are no longer able to keep up with their workload. Waste products build up in your blood. Your kidneys will finally stop working. Kidney dialysis or a kidney transplant are required to remove the toxins from your body.

Do your best to get your blood glucose levels nearer to normal, exercise, and choose healthy meals. Your doctor may ask you to cut back on salty foods and protein. Drink plenty of water every day. And think positive about your health and future.

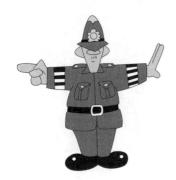

*H*ow *can I reduce my risk of kidney complications?*

**K**eeping your blood glucose under control is the best way to prevent diabetes complications. There are ways to keep tabs on how your kidneys are doing and keep them healthy. You should:

- Have a urine test to check for microalbumin every year if you have type 2 diabetes and after you have had type 1 for more than five years. Be sure it's a microalbumin test and not an ordinary test for urine protein (this does not show microalbumin). Using 24-hour urine collection is the most accurate test, but that's not always necessary.
- If you have microalbuminuria, with or without high blood pressure, use an ACE inhibitor to protect your kidneys from damage.
- Control high blood pressure, even mild high blood pressure. The recommended blood pressure goal is 130/80. ACE inhibitors treat high blood pressure and have a beneficial effect on your kidneys.
- Follow your doctor's advice about how much protein and salt to eat.
- Don't smoke.

*I*'ve heard something about "male menopause." Does it exist and will it affect my diabetes?

▼
## TIP:

What you've heard about is called andropause, and like menopause, it is caused by a drop in hormone levels—testosterone instead of estrogen. It also occurs in men in their 40s and 50s. However, andropause is more subtle and less predictable. Some of the symptoms include:

- Low sex drive
- Fatigue or loss of energy
- Emotional, psychological, and behavioral changes
- Decreased muscle mass and loss of muscle strength
- Increased upper- and central-body fat
- Reduced bone density

Luckily, there is no direct association between diabetes and andropause. However, unrecognized and untreated andropause can cause you to gain weight and increase your risk for diabetes-related problems. The solution is to add more activity to your daily schedule and to eat wisely. You can increase your muscle mass and strength and retain bone density by doing weight-bearing exercises, such as walking or lifting small weights. This will help with your diabetes control, too.

If you think you're suffering from andropause, talk to your physician. Treatment with testosterone replacement therapy may be beneficial.

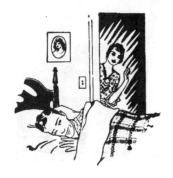

*I've been having problems with impotence. Is it from getting older or from diabetes?*

## ▼ TIP:

Yes, diabetes-related damage to nerves and circulation can cause impotence but so can aging. Impotence is not unique to diabetes. Millions of men who don't have diabetes do have impotence, and frequently the cause is psychological. Sexual enjoyment requires a healthy connection between brain and penis, and a physical shortcoming may not always be the problem. Impotence related to diabetes, on the other hand, has possible physical causes. The more common ones are:

- Nerve damage (neuropathy)
- Reduction of blood flow to the penis (made worse by smoking)
- Low levels of testosterone (the male sex hormone)
- Medications—pills for high blood pressure, anxiety, depression, and peptic ulcer (Don't stop taking your medications without your doctor's approval.)
- Drinking too much alcohol

There are tests available to help determine the causes of impotence. Talk with your doctor about your concern and your options for treatment. Get your blood sugar under control now to keep your sexual health in top form.

*I*f I have impotence caused by
diabetes, how can I treat it?

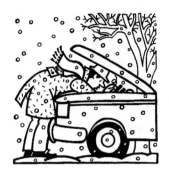

▼
# TIP:

The best way to prevent diabetes-related impotence is
with good blood glucose control, exercise, and by not
smoking. But diabetes may not be the cause. Treatments
depend on the cause and include:

- Working with a therapist to overcome impotence based on
  psychological issues.
- Medication injected or inserted into the penis.
- A cylindrical vacuum pump into which the penis is placed,
  and from which air is pumped out, creating a negative pressure and pulling blood into the penis. Placing a rubber band
  at the base of the penis maintains the erection.
- Testosterone therapy, if testosterone levels are low.
- A variety of oral medications, such as Viagra, intended to
  create an erection.
- Checking to see which of your other medications, such as
  pills for high blood pressure or anti-depressants, could be
  causing impotence and seeing if another drug will work
  better for you.

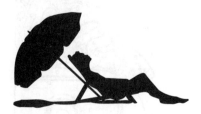

# $W$ill menopause affect my diabetes?

▼
## TIP:

$Y$es. Unpredictable swings in hormones (estrogen and progesterone) affect your blood glucose levels during puberty, pregnancy, menstruation, and menopause. Menopause is when production of estrogen and progesterone slows and finally stops. It usually occurs between the ages of 45 and 55 but may be sooner or later in life.

Estrogen and progesterone counteract the effects of insulin in your body, so when they are high, your blood glucose may also be high. When levels of these hormones fall, your blood glucose may be lower than you expect, and you may be surprised by hypoglycemia. If you use insulin or diabetes pills, you may need to decrease the dose. You may need to check your blood glucose levels more often than usual when you are going through a time of hot flashes and other symptoms of menopause.

Be aware that estrogen provides protection to your heart, and you lose that protection during menopause. Take care to take care of your heart (see tips on pages 14 and 75).

*Since I have diabetes, should I take hormones at menopause?*

▼
## TIP:

Maybe. Diabetes puts you at high risk for heart disease, and that risk increases when your body stops making estrogen. Hormone replacement therapy (HRT) with estrogen and progesterone is sometimes recommended. HRT is not advised if you have a history of breast or uterine cancer, blood clotting problems, severe eye disease, or kidney disease. You may want to try it if you have family history of heart disease or osteoporosis or if you have high cholesterol. If you take HRT, your doctor must monitor your blood fats closely. Another point is that women who take hormones are more likely to have gallbladder problems, which is also a common problem for people with diabetes.

On the plus side is that HRT helps with vaginal dryness, loss of desire, and other menopause-related sexual problems. Weigh the pros and cons of HRT with your doctor. Newer forms of estrogen and progesterone may have fewer side effects and fewer health risks for women with diabetes. Also, you may want to add soy foods to your diet because they contain natural estrogen for your heart and your uncomfortable symptoms.

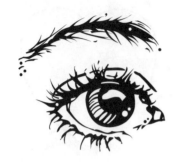 *D oes diabetes affect a woman's ability to enjoy sex?*

## ▼ TIP:

It may, but all women share the following common problems at any and all ages.
Here are the problems and some suggested remedies:

- **Vaginal dryness.** Restore hormone levels if they are low. Use vaginal lubricants if you choose not to use HRT.
- **Pain accompanying sexual intercourse.** Speak to your physician about muscle exercises. Try different positions for intercourse.
- **Vaginal yeast infection.** Control your blood glucose and use medication for the infection. Don't use anything but water to wash your vagina.
- **Nerve damage** in the genital area. A gentle touch or vibration in touch may help.
- **Bladder weakness** (or neurogenic bladder). Always empty your bladder before and after sexual intercourse. Do kegel exercises by stopping the flow of urine midstream and tightening those same muscles at other times (50 kegels a day). Ask your doctor if you should use antibiotics after intercourse to prevent bladder infection.
- **Limited mobility or discomfort** (from neuropathy or arthritis). Vary position or use pillows for support.

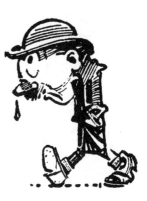

*I*'ve been feeling very depressed lately. Someone mentioned that this could be caused by my diabetes. Is this true?

▼
## TIP:

Y es. If your blood sugar is not being controlled properly, you can suffer from mood swings, confusion, forgetfulness, and most dramatically, depression. Unfortunately, many seniors with diabetes suffer from depression but don't attribute it to their diabetes. If you have any of the following symptoms, talk to your doctor about how to improve your mood:

- Persistent feelings of sadness and emptiness
- Change in sleeping patterns—too much or too little
- Change in appetite
- Lack of desire to do the things you once enjoyed, such as reading, hobbies, and visiting with friends and family
- Extreme fatigue or lack of energy
- Feelings of worthlessness or undeserved guilt

Fortunately, depression can be helped, and if your diabetes is at fault, getting your blood sugar under control can bring some very positive changes. Exercise will improve your mood. There are medications that can make you feel well enough to get up and go—don't wait.

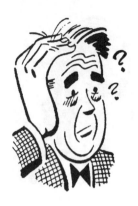

*C*an diabetes cause me to be forgetful and confused?

Yes it can. A lot of seniors with diabetes think that being absentminded and forgetful is just part of the aging process. While some short-term memory loss is expected with aging, there's also a good chance your diabetes is playing a part. High blood sugar can cause you to be, among other things, forgetful, confused, and disoriented. Before blaming a little senility on the years, talk with your doctor about the possibility of high blood sugar.

Try to keep your wits in shape by doing crossword puzzles or playing games, such as Scrabble, chess, or bridge. Research shows that bridge is especially helpful! Try to keep learning new things, such as how to play a musical instrument or speak another language. Every time you learn something new, you create new pathways in your brain that improve your memory and thinking. It makes your life more interesting and you a more interesting person, too.

# Chapter 6
# CHECKUPS THAT COUNT

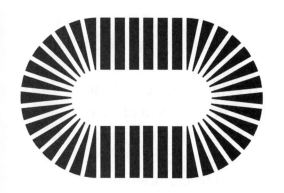

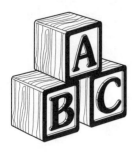

*W*hat do I need to do now that my diabetes has been discovered?

## TIP:

The ADA recommends the following medical help for you:

- A complete medical history and a physical examination that focuses on body "parts" affected by uncontrolled diabetes.
- Laboratory tests: fasting blood fat levels, creatinine (a blood test of kidney function), urinalysis, a urine test for "microalbumin" (trace amounts of protein), a urine culture if infection is suspected, a thyroid function test (for people with type 1 diabetes), and an electrocardiogram.
- A management plan—the key to success with diabetes. This plan takes all things into consideration—your age, lifestyle, daily schedule, physical activity, personality, cultural factors, family, friends, the presence of other health conditions, food preferences, how often you want to check blood glucose, and what your goals are. This plan is the product of discussion between you, your family or friends, and your physician. But you have the final say.
- A schedule for your periodic return visits.

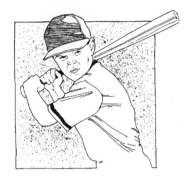

# $W$hat is my HbA1c level?

▼
## TIP:

$H$emoglobin (Hb) is a protein in your blood that carries oxygen from the lungs to tissues. HbA1c is a type of hemoglobin (type A), and when glucose attaches to it, it becomes HbA1c. So why is it important to you? Because your HbA1c level tells you your average blood glucose level for the past two to three months. It's your blood sugar "batting average," and it lets you know how well you're managing your diabetes.

Hemoglobin is packaged in red blood cells. Red blood cells live for 100–120 days, and during this period, the hemoglobin gets a coating of the glucose that's circulating in your blood. By measuring the percentage of sugar-coated HbA1c cells in your blood, you can determine the average amount of glucose that has been in your blood for the previous two or three months.

A normal HbA1c is 4–6.4%. The goal of diabetes management in most people is to have an HbA1c closer to normal levels, about 7%, depending on your health and age. Research has shown clearly that this is the way you can prevent or slow development of long-term complications of diabetes. Check with your doctor to see what your HbA1c is.

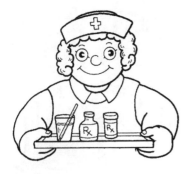

*W*ho can teach me how to use a blood glucose meter?

▼
## TIP:

To be sure, individual or group instruction is the best way to learn. Consider the following possibilities:

- A doctor with interest in diabetes management usually has an assistant skilled in meter education.
- The local hospital may have a diabetes teaching program.
- There may be a diabetes nurse educator working alone or with a physician in your community.
- The pharmacist who sells meters or test strips may have a special knowledge and interest in meter use.
- If all else fails, ask for advice from the nearest American Diabetes Association office.
- Blood glucose meters all have an instruction booklet. Everything you need to know is there. You can also call the company for guidance. Company resources are available online, too.

And remember—experience is the best teacher. You will learn much in doing it. After a year or two, take a refresher course, just to be sure you're still doing it right.

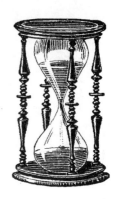

*H*ow often should I check my blood
glucose?

*I*t depends on how stable your diabetes is. People with type 2
diabetes usually have smaller swings in glucose than people
with type 1 diabetes. If you are challenged by wide swings in
glucose, you might want to check four to eight times daily.
People on tight control do. If you have a stable glucose pattern, you would check perhaps every two or three days.

It is important to check not only in the morning or before
meals, but also 1–2 hours after meals, and perhaps during the
night. You could spread these checks out over the week so that
you always do a morning fasting check and one other at a
different time each day.

Routines in life help you have a stable and healthy
existence. Checking your glucose level is an important part of
your routine. It gives you information and confidence and
security.

Many meters store the results. But you also need information about the date, time, meals, events, exercise, and
medication. You would benefit from keeping a log book of
this information that you can take to doctor's appointments.
You use this information to decide when to eat, how much to
eat, when to exercise, and how much diabetes medication to
take.

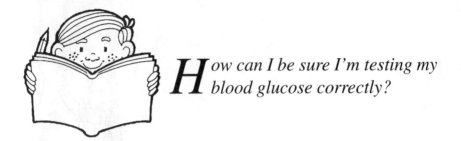

*H*ow can I be sure I'm testing my blood glucose correctly?

▼
## TIP:

The top testing tips are:

- Use the instruction manual to check your technique.
- Select a meter that meets your needs, say with a larger display screen or audio readings.
- Use the side of any finger. Do not use the center of the fingertip because it will hurt more. Some use areas other than a finger, for example the forearm.
- Keep the sensor and strip areas of the meter clean.
- Be sure that the meter is properly calibrated on a schedule.
- Periodically check your meter's accuracy (and your technique) with a control solution.
- Your meter should be accurate to within 15% of your doctor's laboratory results, and this is okay for your use.
- If blood flows slowly, warm your hands before taking the sample.
- Make sure your hands are dry with no soap still on them.
- Don't fret about the number. Just use it to decide what to do.

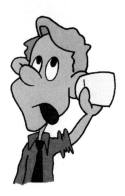

*I* *can't see well. How can I test my glucose?*

# TIP:

S everal glucose meters can be equipped to give step-by-step verbal instructions for testing and to report the results audibly. English is the standard language, but other languages are available. Additional features available with selected talking meters include cassette instructions, Braille identification of controls, and plug-in ports, earphones, and large print instructions. At least one device reads the bar codes on the insulin bottles and verbally identifies the insulin contained in the bottle, so you don't make a mistake getting the right one. In all cases, the synthesized voice is considerate and non-judgmental. Ask your doctor, diabetes educator, or pharmacist for help finding a system that is comfortable for you.

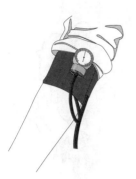

# $W$hat should my blood pressure be?

$F$or good health, blood pressure should be no more than 130/80. Setting the goal at 130/80 or below is a reasonable and safe objective. Controlling your blood pressure is the way to reduce your risk of developing diabetes-related complications and other serious health conditions, such as having a stroke.

The first and most important steps to take control of high blood pressure are lifestyle changes. These include losing weight, exercising more, reducing the amount of salt (sodium) you eat (read the food labels), and limiting the amount of alcohol you drink.

If lifestyle changes do not bring your blood pressure down, your doctor will prescribe medication for it. If one medication doesn't do the job, another, and perhaps another are added in a stepwise fashion (see page 31). Blood pressure pills have side effects, so be sure you understand what they are.

# W*hat is a lipid?*

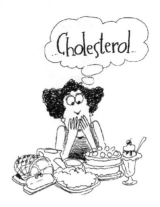

▼
## TIP:

Lipids are blood fats. There are different kinds of lipids, and they form important structural parts of the human body. However, several kinds of lipids are linked to hardening of the arteries (atherosclerosis). If you eat meals that are high in saturated fat, and are very overweight and physically inactive, you have the ingredients for lipid problems.

There are three kinds of blood fats that affect blood vessels—HDL cholesterol (good cholesterol), LDL cholesterol, and triglycerides. To maintain health, try to keep your lipid levels as follows:

- HDL cholesterol protects against atherosclerosis. Blood test values less than 35 mg/dl are unhealthy. Values above 45 mg/dl in men and above 55 mg/dl in women are healthy.
- LDL cholesterol should be at low levels to reduce the risk of atherosclerosis. Levels above 130 mg/dl carry risk. Values below 100 mg/dl are healthy.
- Triglycerides should be at levels below 200 mg/dl. Increased levels are linked to inflammation of the pancreas (pancreatitis), and are likely involved in atherosclerosis.

Have your lipids tested every year to make sure you're maintaining healthy levels of blood fats.

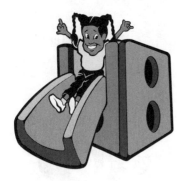

*H* *ow do I control my lipids, and why?*

Y ou control lipids to save your heart. You reduce your chance of developing coronary heart disease (heart trouble from "hardening" of the arteries that nourish the heart). If you already have coronary heart disease, lipid control will reduce the chance of it getting worse.

There are four cornerstones of lipid control.

- A meal plan. A meal plan for glucose control will improve certain lipid disorders. Fats in a meal plan are more unsaturated fats (olive or canola oils) than saturated (animal products). Too much alcohol may cause irregularity of certain lipids, so it's wise to cut back.
- Weight reduction. When you cut back your total daily calories by eating less fat (the high-calorie foodstuff), you lose weight.
- Physical activity. Increasing your physical activity will, by itself, improve lipid levels and aid in successful weight loss.
- If your lipids are not in good control after 3–6 months of cornerstone therapy, you may need a medication—the type depends on the type of lipid disorder.

*I can't move much, how can I take care of my feet?*

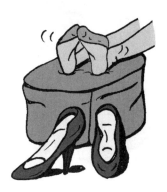

▼
# TIP:

Try these tips:

- Get a bench or stool for your bathtub or shower, so you can sit to clean your feet.
- Have grab bars installed in your shower, so you can support yourself when you bend over.
- Buy or make a long-handled sponge or bath brush, so you can wash your feet.
- Lay a towel on the floor, and rub your feet across the towel to dry them (try to dry well between the toes).
- Have another long-handled sponge or brush to apply lotion (do not use the same one you use in the shower).
- To inspect the bottom of your feet, lay a mirror on the floor and hold your foot above it to see underneath.
- Ask your spouse or a friend to inspect the bottom of your feet for you.
- Never go barefoot, unless you are bathing or sleeping.
- If you lose feeling in your feet, have your doctor look at them at each visit.

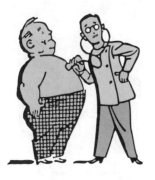

*W*hat medical tests should I get
to take care of my diabetes?

▼
## TIP:

Continuing care is important. The ADA recommends:

- Doctor visits whenever needed. If you need changes in treatment, visits may be daily or weekly. If all is stable, then your visits are every 3–6 months.
- At each visit, give a recent medical history and get a physical examination.
- At each visit, your diabetes plan should be reviewed and adjusted, if it's not working for you.
- Every 3–6 months, HbA1c should be measured (how often depends on how stable your diabetes control is).
- Yearly, have a complete eye examination, with eye drops to dilate the eyes, performed by an ophthalmologist or optometrist trained in diabetes care.
- Yearly, have a complete foot examination. If you have a risk of foot problems, this examination should be done at every visit.
- Yearly, have a fasting lipid blood test if your lipids are in control. If you are at low risk, every two years is okay. You need blood tests more often when lipids are out of control.
- Yearly, have a urine test for microalbumin. If your urine contains albumin, and therapy is prescribed to control it, you may be tested more often.

# Chapter 7
# DOCTORS, NURSES, AND YOU

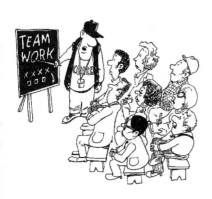

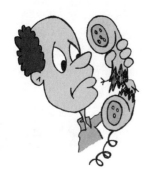

*M*y doctor acts like he doesn't have time to talk to me; what can I do?

▼
## TIP:

Your doctor is your teammate. To win you must communicate with respect, genuineness, good manners, and unconditional acceptance. Beware the pitfalls that stud the playing field for both of you. Does your doctor want to control the conversation by asking questions that let you make only "Yes" or "No" answers? Or does he just not have any time?

With a chronic disease, you are the one in charge, and you need the benefit of your doctor's knowledge, both clinical facts and personal expertise. Write down your questions before you go so you are organized and use the appointed time well. Ask him to refer you to a diabetes educator, so you can learn more about diabetes in a more relaxed setting.

Learn to speak up for yourself. The doctor serves as an active guide, but he needs the information that only you have about you. Once you have been fully informed, you set your own goals. If you are truly frustrated that you are not being heard or helped, then you may have to change doctors.

# $H$ *ow can I make a doctor's visit go smoothly?*

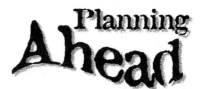

▼
## TIP:

- Be sure you understand what your doctor is saying! If you have trouble hearing, say so. Ask him or her to speak up or write his directions for you.
- Respect the time allowed for your visit. There is a limit to the number of issues you can discuss. Prepare a list of the most important issues.
- Inform the doctor's secretary of insurance changes or need to have paperwork done.
- Bring a list of your medications and doses (or bring the bottles). Have your glucose log book open for review.
- Inform the doctor of lifestyle (exercise, for example) or meal plan changes.
- Wear clothing that is easy to remove.
- Don't bring the family. A friend or your spouse may be important, but a group of people spreads chaos.
- Request help from the doctor's staff with removal of clothing or getting on the examining table.
- Be sure to get lab tests done far enough ahead so that results are available at the visit.
- You may call or email between appointments, but don't discuss major issues that way.
- Accept that your doctor is human, too. Smile.
- Not working? Change doctors.

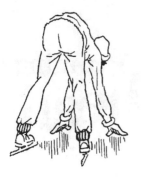

*W*ho should make the final decisions,
the patient or the doctor?

▼
## TIP:

*I*t is your life. It is your decision.

Forty years ago, Bill developed diabetes at age 36. At 76, he has enjoyed a rich quality of life, but time has taken its toll. Kidney malfunction has required kidney dialysis three times weekly over the past five years. Strong in mind, he is physically enfeebled by years and circumstances. Although his physician is anxious to carry on with dialysis, Bill wants to stop and spend the final days at home with his family.

There is a beginning and there is an end to all things. Reaching the older side of age often brings dilemmas in what to do and how much to do for health care. Advances in technology have brought amazing treatment options. But what do you do when continuing treatment no longer brings quality of life? An informed person of sound mind has the privilege of deciding what is best. Final days spent with family and other loved ones, spent on unfinished business, spent in peace, can be the most meaningful days of a person's life.

Bill will be making his decision soon. It's the right one.

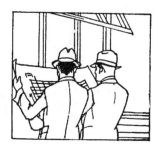

*W*hat should my medical insurance cover in diabetes care?

▼
## TIP:

Your insurance should cover the check-ups and tests you need to stay healthy. You should be able to see your doctor regularly (four times a year for type 1 and one or two times a year for type 2) and get your HbA1c, blood pressure, and blood fats (if necessary) checked. You should also have yearly dilated eye exams. These checkups benefit your health and well-being, reduce the complications of diabetes, and significantly reduce health care costs. ADA believes that health insurers must cover the following:

- health care visits
- diabetes education by a trained team
- laboratory tests as needed
- all medications and supplies for complete diabetes care

However, not all insurance will cover all these areas. In recent years, progress has been made on state and national levels, both in government and private insurance companies. But as you know, reimbursement is spotty. The health care dollar is only so big. Join the cause to make others more aware! Lobby your lawmakers and insurance company for what we believe is your right. Be in touch with the ADA and find out how you can help in securing proper reimbursement for all people with diabetes.

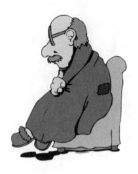

*I live in a nursing home and seem to catch a lot of colds. How do I manage diabetes when I am sick?*

▼
## TIP:

Your doctor or educator should help you make a sick-day plan ahead of time. Glucose levels vary during illness but usually are high. Key points are:

- Frequent blood glucose checks, four times or more daily, to see where your glucose level is.
- If glucose is above 240 mg/dl, check your urine for ketones. Ketones alert you to developing ketoacidosis.
- If you take diabetes medications, continue to take them on schedule. Insulin, or extra insulin, may be required temporarily if your glucose is too high. Take a little even if you can't keep food down. This is important.
- If you're nauseated or vomiting, drinking small amounts (2–4 oz) of regular (not diet) soda or juice every 2–3 hours is usually easier on your stomach. Getting some carbohydrate is important for energy. Eat food that is easy on your stomach, such as crackers or broth.
- Manage the illness as well as the diabetes.
- Set guidelines ahead of time for when to call your physician. Be able to tell him what your blood glucose level is, your temperature, and your ketone level.

# Chapter 8
# SHARPENING YOUR WITS

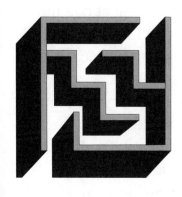

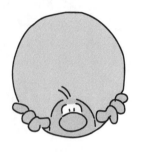

*I*'m not as hungry any more, and I eat
less often. Will this affect my diabetes
control?

▼
**TIP:**

Yes. This is a change in your meal plan. If you use insulin,
sulfonylureas, or Prandin, not eating can put you at risk
for very low blood sugar (hypoglycemia). Eating at odd times
may give you wide swings in blood sugar and malnutrition.
We do need less food as we age, but we still need to eat to
stay healthy.

Perhaps you cannot taste or smell the food. Try brushing
your tongue as well as your teeth before you eat. Stop
smoking to improve your senses. Eat more fresh foods and
use herbs and spices for flavor instead of salt.

Could you be depressed? Clinical depression is common in
diabetes and certainly affects your appetite. Talk with your
doctor about your symptoms. When you are depressed, it's
difficult to be interested in doing things for yourself or staying
healthy. It can keep you from getting up and going for a walk.

Getting exercise will help build your appetite, improve
your mental outlook, and give you more energy.

*H*<sup></sup>*ow do I let go?*

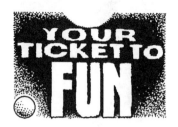

▼
## TIP:

R ealize that "He who laughs, lasts." Yes, diabetes is hard work and frustrating at times. There are situations and events that just cannot be explained or resolved. In tough times, humor can be the great healer. It releases tension, lowers your blood pressure, and makes you healthier all over.

Jane received a Lilly 60-Year Medal at age 78. She has outlived two husbands—who were worriers, far too serious. She was using intensive therapy 60 years ago. Insulin was available only in rapid-acting murky brown solution, and she injected it four times daily with large re-sharpened hypo-dermic needles attached to glass syringes that she boiled periodically and stored in alcohol. She has developed some complications of diabetes over the decades, but she is knowl-edgeable, proud, and graceful. What has supported her is humor. She jokes about her limitations and puts her physi-cians at ease if they are struggling to figure out her diabetes care plan. Her appreciation for and use of humor allows her to live a full and productive life.

Work hard, and let go just as hard. Try to laugh at least once every day!

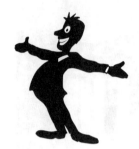

*I'm in my 70s. Should I be concerned about target blood glucose levels?*

Yes. Effective glucose control improves health at any age. However, you may need to have higher target glucose levels. They should be higher if you:

- Take diabetes medications, including insulin, at incorrect times. Your blood glucose levels could go dangerously low.
- Eat at irregular times.
- Have had a stroke or reduced brain circulation. You may not recognize the symptoms of falling glucose and get into trouble.
- Live alone. It may be hard to get help when you have falling blood glucose.
- Have gastroparesis. This fancy word means "sluggish stomach function," and is a type of neuropathy. The food you eat may not be processed speedily and your glucose levels may be up or down at unexpected times.
- Have neuropathy. In this condition, you may no longer have any symptoms of falling glucose.
- Exercise. Exercise lowers glucose during and for hours after the activity, so you may have a higher level before (not above 250 mg/dl), so you don't go too low afterward.

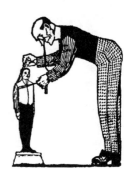

*H*ow much weight do I have to lose to
control diabetes?

If you have type 2 diabetes, you probably weigh more than
you should, or did when you were diagnosed. If this is the
case, the first thing your physician probably told you was,
"Lose some weight!" It's a tough job, but it's essential to
getting your diabetes under control.

So, how much weight is enough to see results? 2 pounds?
10 pounds? 150? Actually, any weight you lose will be
beneficial. But to see real results, a loss of 10–20 pounds can
do wonders and can be accomplished in 3 to 4 months. Not
only will your blood glucose levels drop (meaning less
medication, which means less expense), but you'll also feel
better, and your risk for other serious health problems will
drop, too.

Losing weight means doing some exercise and changing
the way you eat. It may be as simple a step as measuring—
with a measuring cup or a scale—each serving that you eat.
Even if it's healthy food, too much is still too much.

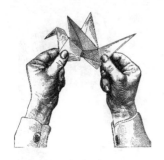

*I'm retired; isn't it time to just sit?*

▼
## TIP:

It isn't healthy for anyone of any age to just sit. For example, Sharon expected an enriched life when she retired from nursing in her early 60s. But she found herself adrift, stressed, preoccupied by petty ailments, gaining weight, inactive, and lacking self worth.

Although health care professionals are usually poor patients, she had the good sense to get a checkup. Her weight, high blood pressure, and family history of diabetes led to blood glucose tests. And in fact, Sharon had high fasting blood glucose on two occasions—diabetes.

She attacked the condition she was in. She began a program of physical fitness. She got a meal plan and followed it. Her weight dropped, and she was able to control her blood glucose without medication. She took a small dose of an ACE inhibitor to control her blood pressure.

Her success in managing the diabetes rekindled her sense of self-worth and put Sharon back on course. In fact, she returned to nursing and continues to work in an office serving the needs of other people with diabetes.

# Chapter 9
# FRIENDS AND FAMILY

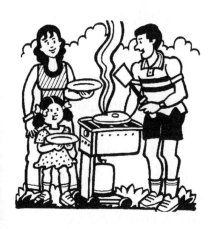

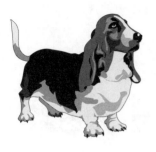

*C*an I manage my diabetes by myself?

It would be best if you would share it. Companionship and personal relationships are important throughout life, and over the years, may become necessary for help in managing your health. It may spell the difference between living independently and having to move from your home.

Companionship can include a spouse, family member, hired caregiver, hospice volunteer, Good Samaritan, or pet. Yes, pets qualify. They are not skilled at administering medications but are good at many tasks and are ideal companions (*Animals are such agreeable friends—they ask no questions, they pass no criticisms.*—George Eliot).

Encourage a companion in your life. A companion can serve many functions beyond the delights of socializing and intellectual stimulation. It is no accident that you are encouraged to bring a companion to most diabetes education programs. With knowledge of diabetes, the companion can help prepare meals, monitor glucose, give medication, and participate in all your activities of daily living. Diabetes is safer.

And remember, the way to have a friend is to be a friend. Encourage and keep good friends. Your life will be much richer, and your diabetes easier to manage.

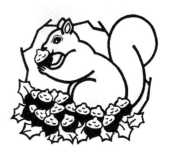

*H*ow can I make things easier for myself and my family if I get very ill?

**P**lan ahead and get the documents, such as a will, written now. Sherm was a fire inspector—he did things by the book. At age 68, he developed raging bone infection in his left foot. Thirty-four years of diabetes has marked him with neuropathy and poor circulation in the legs. This bone infection had happened before and required partial amputation of the left foot. This time, he didn't want surgery and was willing to accept whatever happened.

Sherm was prepared. All adults should plan and make known their end-of-life decisions. Such planning is a service to your family and friends. Sherm had the following documents properly completed:

- Will
- Advance directive—stating his personal wishes regarding being given CPR, IV feedings, and other interventions, which is to be used if he is unable to make such decisions when they are needed
- Durable power of attorney—assigning decision-making authority regarding his health care to a designated person, a person who knows his wishes and who will act on his behalf if and when he is unable to make such decisions

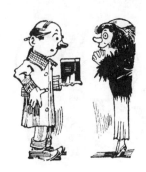

*W*hy did my wife's personality really change after she got diabetes?

## ▼ TIP:

It would take a book to answer, but let's start with questions that can apply to anyone with diabetes. Personality doesn't very often change. What was her personality before diabetes? What was your relationship before diabetes? Is the household one of harmony and understanding? Diabetes causes stress and threatens stability. Has diabetes changed your expectations or lifestyle? Are you supportive and understanding? Is your lifestyle healthy, or do you resent making the changes that are important for her?

Is she keeping it all in and not talking about it? Is she overwhelmed by fear? Does she need the confidence that comes from diabetes education? Is she frustrated by her relationship with her doctors? Is she worried or guilty about the possibility of passing diabetes to your children or grandchildren? Is she afraid of letting you down? Is she clinically depressed? Is she in one of the five stages of grief—denial, anger, bargaining, depression, or acceptance?

Diabetes is a challenge, often creating emotional turmoil. But with support from you and her health care providers, she can manage her diabetes with a smile most of the time.

Try to lighten the mood every day. Compliment her. And share laughter—it's still the best medicine.

*H* ow do I manage large meals at special celebrations?

▼
## TIP:

S pecial celebrations are an important part of our culture. Here are some tips to remain popular and avoid frustration, weight gain, and poor glucose control:

- Stay confident and in control. It's okay to be who you are.
- Remember that all foods can fit your meal plan in reasonable amounts—even 2 bites of your favorite dessert.
- Don't change your usual eating pattern, except you might omit snacks that day.
- Be proud of your discipline. Focus on the event and not on the food and drink.
- Honor the host and hostess. Smile, accept what you're served graciously, and limit the amounts of food you eat (you won't be the only one doing this).
- Ask to take a portion home to eat tomorrow.
- Be prepared. Discuss these situations ahead of time with your doctor and dietician and have a plan. If you take insulin, you may take extra rapid-acting insulin to cover more carbohydrate in the meal. Meglitinide pills can be adjusted just before meals as needed. People using other oral medications may use supplemental insulin for situations such as this.

*I don't know anything about cooking. Who's going to cook if my wife is sick?*

▼
# TIP:

You can do it. Sure, you could eat out every night, but a home-cooked meal is healthier and can express creativity and love. It pays back some of what you've received over the years. If you're new to the kitchen (and maybe a little overwhelmed), keep these things in mind:

- Start with some easy dishes that you like.
- Purchase an ADA cookbook and try new things.
- Watch a cooking show on television for ideas.
- Purchase some new cooking tools to replace or enhance the tools already in your kitchen (your wife may grumble over the fact that you consider hers inferior equipment).
- Take a cooking course and learn to prepare foods you never thought you could cook. You're young as long as you keep learning new things.

It can be as simple as oatmeal for breakfast, a chef salad for lunch, and roast beef with vegetables for dinner. You don't even have to "cook" much. You'll be surprised at how satisfying preparing a good meal can be. Even more rewarding will be the pleasure and appreciation you receive from your wife.

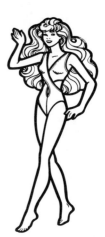

*M*y friends are going on a trendy new diet.
Is it safe for me?

**M**ost likely, the answer is no. There are a lot of new diets that promise rapid weight loss but most do not follow the healthy eating guidelines set up by our government nor those for people with diabetes. When you have diabetes, what you eat is an essential part of your diabetes management plan. Not following your meal plan could lead to poor health for you. In fact, many of these diets can be hard on your body and deprive you of nutrients that you need.

When all is said and done, the only diet that works is one that restricts the number of calories eaten in a day and adds exercise to your daily routine. You'll do better to design a meal plan that fits your needs and lifestyle with an RD. You take weight off slowly over time and that's the best way to do it—with a good balanced meal plan to keep you healthy throughout the process. When your friends are back to where they started, you'll be glad you did it your way.

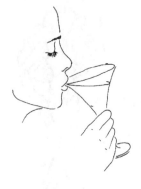

*I enjoy a drink every once in awhile and have for over 50 years. Is diabetes going to force me to give up my evening cocktail?*

It doesn't have to. In fact, an occasional drink, such as a glass of wine with dinner, can have health benefits both mental and physical. However, there are precautions to take when drinking alcoholic beverages:

- Limit daily drinks to two for men and one for women. One drink equals 12 oz beer, 5 oz wine, or 1½ oz distilled spirits.
- Fit the alcohol into your daily meal plan. It has lots of calories. One alcoholic beverage equals two fat exchanges. Beer, sweet wines, and mixers contain additional carbohydrate and calories that will affect your blood sugar level—and maybe your weight.
- If you don't eat food when you are having the drink, alcohol can cause very low levels of blood glucose (hypoglycemia). This is especially dangerous since low blood glucose and drunkenness have similar symptoms. While people are figuring out that you are not drunk, there may be a serious delay in getting the treatment you need to raise your blood sugar.
- Never drink and drive.

# Chapter 10
# RESOURCES

# Books from the ADA

*101 Medication Tips for People with Diabetes* by Mary Anne Koda-Kimble, PharmD, CDE; Betsy A. Carlisle, PharmD; and Lisa A. Kroon, PharmD

*101 Tips for Improving Your Blood Sugar,* 2nd edition, by David S. Schade, MD, and associates

*101 Tips for Staying Healthy with Diabetes (& Avoiding Complications*), 2nd edition, by David S. Schade, MD, and associates

*101 Nutrition Tips for People with Diabetes* by Patti B. Geil, MS, RD, FADA, CDE; and Lea Ann Holzmeister, RD, CDE

*101 Foot Care Tips for People with Diabetes* by Jesse H. Ahroni, PhD, ARNP, CDE

*The "I Hate to Exercise" Book for People with Diabetes* by Charlotte Hayes, MMSc, MS, RD, CDE

*Diabetes Burnout: What to Do When You Can't Take It Anymore* by William H. Polonsky, PhD, CDE (also available on audio tape)

*The Diabetes Travel Guide* by Davida F. Kruger, MSN, RN, CS, CDE

*Women & Diabetes: Staying Healthy in Body, Mind, and Spirit* by Laurinda M Poirier, RN, MPH, CDE; and Katherine M. Coburn, MPH

*Mr. Food's Quick & Easy Diabetic Cooking* by Art Ginsberg with Miss America 1999, Nicole Johnson

*ADA Complete Guide to Carb Counting* by Hope Warshaw, MMSc, RD, CDE; and Karmeen Kulkarni, MS, RD, CDE

## Exercise Videos

**Armchair Fitness Videos**
(800) 453-6280
web site: www.ArmchairFitness.com

**Lilias! Flowing Postures Series**
**Lilias! Yoga Workout for Beginners**
**Lilias! Silver Yoga Series**
(800) 250-8760
Also available in Target, Wal-Mart, and other stores that sell videos.

## For People over 50

**American Association for Retired Persons (AARP)**
601 E Street, NW
Washington, DC 20049
(202) 434-2277
(800) 456-2277 (pharmacy)
(202) 434-2558 (fax)
(800) 424-3410 (membership)
web site: *http://www.aarp.org*

## National Council on the Aging
409 3rd Street, 2nd Floor
Washington, DC 20024
(800) 424-9047
(202) 479-1200
(202) 479-0735 (fax)


## For the Visually Challenged

### American Council of the Blind
1155 15th Street, NW, Suite 720
Washington, DC  20005
(202) 467-5081
(800) 424-8666
(202) 331-1058
e-mail: *ncrabb@acb.org*
web site: *http://www.acb.org*

### American Foundation for the Blind
11 Penn Plaza, Suite 300
New York, NY  10001
(212) 502-7600
(800) 232-5463
e-mail: *asbinfo@asb.org*
internet: *gopher.asb.org_5005*

# For Amputees

**American Amputee Foundation**
PO Box 250218
Little Rock, AR 72225
(501) 666-2523
(501) 666-8367 (fax)

# For Those Needing Long-term or Home Care

**National Association for Home Care (NHAC)**
228 7th Street SE
Washington, DC 20003
(202) 547-7424
(202) 547-3540 (fax)
web site: *http://www.nahc.org*

**Nursing Home Information Service**
c/o National Council of Senior Citizens
8403 Colesville Road, Suite 1200
Silver Spring, MD 20910
(301) 578-8800, ext. 8839
(301) 578-8999 (fax)

# For Travelers

**International Association for Medical Assistance to Travelers**
417 Center Street
Lewiston, NY 14092
(716) 754-4883
(519) 836-3412 (fax)

# For Insurance Information

**Social Security Administration**
(800) 772-1213

**Medicare Hotline**
(800) 638-6833

**Medicare Publications**
Health Care Financing Administration
6325 Security Boulevard
Baltimore, MD 21207

# For Miscellaneous Health Information

**American Association of Diabetes Educators**
444 North Michigan Avenue, Suite 1240
Chicago, IL 60611
(312) 644-2233
(800) 832-6874
(312) 644-4411 (fax)

**American Heart Association**
7272 Greenville Avenue
Dallas, TX 75231
(800) 242-8721
website: *http://www.amhrt.org*

# INDEX

**M**
Magnesium deficiency, 33
Male menopause
  see Andropause
Medication, 21, 28, 34, 72
Meglitinides, 21, 22, 23, 51
Memory, 78
Menopause, 74
Metformin, 21, 22, 23
Microalbumin, 69, 70, 90
Miglitol, 21
Minerals, 33
Monoamine oxidase inhibitors (MAOs), 28
Monofilament, 63

**N**
Nephropathy, 50, 69
Neurogenic bladder, 76
Neuropathy, 50, 53, 65, 66, 72, 76, 100
  autonomic, 67
  distal symmetrical polyneuropathy, 67
  entrapment, 67
  peripheral, 62, 68
Nicotinic acid, 28
Nursing home, 13

**O**
Occupational therapist, 27, 35
Ophthalmologist, 61
Organization, 16, 17, 34
Osteoporosis, 55

**P**
Personality change, 77, 78, 106
Phenothiazines, 28
Phenytoin, 28
Physical examination, 80, 90
Physicians, working with, 92, 93
Pills, 21, 22, 23, 24, 31
  cutting of, 29
Pioglitazone, 21
Pneumonia vaccine, 32
Potassium, 33
Prandin, 21, 22, 28

Prednisone, 28
Pseudoephedrine, 28

**R**
Registered dietician (RD), 37, 43, 109
Repaglinide, 21
Resources, 18
Retinopathy, 50, 53, 60, 61, 68
Retiring, 102
Rosiglitazone, 21

**S**
Sex drive,
  in men, 71, 72
  in women, 75, 76
Sluggish stomach function
  see Gastroparesis
Smoking, 14, 37, 50, 55, 66, 70, 72, 73
Stroke, 58, 86
Sugar, 39
Sulfonylureas, 21, 22, 23, 28, 51
Syringe magnifiers, 27

**T**
Testosterone, 55, 71, 72, 73
Thiazide diuretics, 31
Thiazolidinediones, 21, 22, 23
Thromboxane, 30
Traveling, 17
Triglyceride, 22, 88
Type 1 diabetes, 5
Type 2 diabetes, 5, 52

**V**
Viagra, 73
Vitamins, 33

**W**
Water, 41
Weight, 54, 101
Will planning, 105

**Y**
Yoga, 52, 53

# About the American Diabetes Association

The American Diabetes Association is the nation's leading voluntary health organization supporting diabetes research, information, and advocacy. Its mission is to prevent and cure diabetes and to improve the lives of all people affected by diabetes. The American Diabetes Association is the leading publisher of comprehensive diabetes information. Its huge library of practical and authoritative books for people with diabetes covers every aspect of self-care—cooking and nutrition, fitness, weight control, medications, complications, emotional issues, and general self-care.

To order American Diabetes Association books: Call 1-800-232-6733. http://store.diabetes.org [Note: there is no need to use www when typing this particular Web address]

To join the American Diabetes Association: Call 1-800-806-7801. www.diabetes.org/membership

For more information about diabetes or ADA programs and services: Call 1-800-342-2383. E-mail: Customerservice@diabetes.org www.diabetes.org

To locate an ADA/NCQA Recognized Provider of quality diabetes care in your area: Call 1-703-549-1500 ext. 2202. www.diabetes.org/recognition/Physicians/ListAll.asp

To find an ADA Recognized Education Program in your area: Call 1-888-232-0822. www.diabetes.org/recognition/education.asp

To join the fight to increase funding for diabetes research, end discrimination, and improve insurance coverage: Call 1-800-342-2383. www.diabetes.org/advocacy

To find out how you can get involved with the programs in your community: Call 1-800-342-2383. See below for program Web addresses.

- American Diabetes Month: Educational activities aimed at those diagnosed with diabetes—month of November. www.diabetes.org/ADM
- American Diabetes Alert: Annual public awareness campaign to find the undiagnosed—held the fourth Tuesday in March. www.diabetes.org/alert
- The Diabetes Assistance & Resources Program (DAR): diabetes awareness program targeted to the Latino community. www.diabetes.org/DAR
- African American Program: diabetes awareness program targeted to the African American community. www.diabetes.org/africanamerican
- Awakening the Spirit: Pathways to Diabetes Prevention & Control: diabetes awareness program targeted to the Native American community. www.diabetes.org/awakening

To find out about an important research project regarding type 2 diabetes: www.diabetes.org/ada/research.asp

To obtain information on making a planned gift or charitable bequest: Call 1-888-700-7029. www.diabetes.org/ada/plan.asp

To make a donation or memorial contribution: Call 1-800-342-2383. www.diabetes.org/ada/cont.asp